The U.S. Health Care Spending: Comparison with Other OECD Countries

THE U.S. HEALTH CARE SPENDING: COMPARISON WITH OTHER OECD COUNTRIES

CHRIS L. PETERSON AND RACHEL BURTON

Nova Science Publishers, Inc.
New York

Copyright © 2008 by Nova Science Publishers, Inc.

All rights reserved. No part of this book may be reproduced, stored in a retrieval system or transmitted in any form or by any means: electronic, electrostatic, magnetic, tape, mechanical photocopying, recording or otherwise without the written permission of the Publisher.

For permission to use material from this book please contact us:
Telephone 631-231-7269; Fax 631-231-8175
Web Site: http://www.novapublishers.com

NOTICE TO THE READER

The Publisher has taken reasonable care in the preparation of this book, but makes no expressed or implied warranty of any kind and assumes no responsibility for any errors or omissions. No liability is assumed for incidental or consequential damages in connection with or arising out of information contained in this book. The Publisher shall not be liable for any special, consequential, or exemplary damages resulting, in whole or in part, from the readers' use of, or reliance upon, this material.

Independent verification should be sought for any data, advice or recommendations contained in this book. In addition, no responsibility is assumed by the publisher for any injury and/or damage to persons or property arising from any methods, products, instructions, ideas or otherwise contained in this publication.

This publication is designed to provide accurate and authoritative information with regard to the subject matter covered herein. It is sold with the clear understanding that the Publisher is not engaged in rendering legal or any other professional services. If legal or any other expert assistance is required, the services of a competent person should be sought. FROM A DECLARATION OF PARTICIPANTS JOINTLY ADOPTED BY A COMMITTEE OF THE AMERICAN BAR ASSOCIATION AND A COMMITTEE OF PUBLISHERS.

LIBRARY OF CONGRESS CATALOGING-IN-PUBLICATION DATA
Peterson, Chris L., 1949-
 The U.S. health care spending : comparison with other OECD countries / Chris L. Peterson and Rachel Burton.
  p. ; cm.
 ISBN 978-1-60456-329-0 (hardcover)
 1. Medical care, Cost of--United States. 2. Medical care, Cost of--OECD countries. I. Burton, Rachel. II. Title. III. Title: US health care spending.
 [DNLM: 1. Health Expenditures--United States. 2. Outcome and Process Assessment (Health Care)--economics--United States. 3. Quality of Health Care--economics--United States. W 74 AA1 P485u 2008]
 RA410.53.P43 2008
 338.4'33621--dc22
                    2007051482

Published by Nova Science Publishers, Inc. ~. New York

Contents

Preface		**ix**
Chapter 1	How Much Does the United States Spend on Health Care?	1
Chapter 2	Why Does the United States Spend so Much on Health Care?	7
Chapter 3	Volume: Do Americans Use Health Care More Often?	9
Chapter 4	Intensity: When Americans Receive Care, Is It More Involved?	13
Chapter 5	Intensity of Hospitalizations	15
Chapter 6	Intensity of Doctor Visits	21
Chapter 7	Intra-National Variation in Intensity	29
Chapter 8	Price: Do Americans Pay More for Health Care Services?	31
Chapter 9	Salaries of Health Professionals	33
Chapter 10	Price of Medical Equipment	39
Chapter 11	Price of Medical Procedures	41
Chapter 12	Price of Pharmaceuticals	43
Chapter 13	Health Care Spending by Type of Service	49
Chapter 14	What Spurs Health Care Prices and Utilization?	53
Chapter 15	Factors that Affect Demand	55

Chapter 16	Age Structure of the Population	57
Chapter 17	Income	59
Chapter 18	Insurance	61
Chapter 19	Tax Treatment	65
Chapter 20	Tastes	67
Chapter 21	Weak Bargaining Power	69
Chapter 22	Factors that Affect Supply	71
Chapter 23	Supplier-Induced Demand	73
Chapter 24	Specialist Care Emphasis	75
Chapter 25	Defensive Medicine	77
Chapter 26	Structure of Health System	79
Chapter 27	What Does the United States Get for Its Health Care Spending?	81
Chapter 28	Wait Times	85
Chapter 29	Self-Reported Health Status	87
Chapter 30	Life Expectancy	89
Chapter 31	Mortality Rates	91
Chapter 32	Medical Errors	97
Chapter 33	Infant Mortality Rates	99
Chapter 34	Does the United States Spend "Too Much" on Health Care?	103
Chapter 35	Conclusion	107
Chapter 36	Health Care Resources	109
Chapter 37	Pharmaceuticals	111
Chapter 38	Health Administration and Insurance	113
Chapter 39	Prices	115
Chapter 40	Population Risk Factors	117
Chapter 41	Quality	119

Chapter 42	**Wait Times**	**121**
Chapter 43	**Health Outcomes**	**123**
References		**125**
Index		**137**

PREFACE

The United States spends more money on health care than any other country in the Organization for Economic Cooperation and Development (OECD). The OECD consists of 30 democracies, most of which are considered the most economically advanced countries in the world.

The OECD data and other research provide some insight as to why health care spending is higher in the United States than in other countries, although many difficult research issues remain. This book presents some of the available data and research and concludes with a summary of study findings.

According to OECD data, the United States spent $6,102 per capita on health care in 2004 — more than double the OECD average and 19.9% more than Luxembourg, the second-highest spending country. In 2004, 15.3% of the U.S. economy was devoted to health care, compared with 8.9% in the average OECD country and 11.6% in second-placed Switzerland.

Why does the United States spend this amount on health care? Economists break health care spending into two parts: price and quantity (which includes the number of visits to health care providers and the intensity of those visits). In terms of quantity, OECD data indicate that the United States has far fewer doctor visits per person compared with the OECD average; for hospitalizations, the United States ranks well below the OECD and is roughly comparable in terms of length of hospital stays. The intensity of service delivery is a different story: the United States uses more of the newest medical technologies and performs several invasive procedures (such as coronary bypasses and angioplasties) more frequently than the average OECD country. In terms of price, the OECD has stated that "there is no doubt that U.S. prices for medical care commodities and services are significantly higher than in other countries and serve as a key determinant of higher overall spending."

What does the United States get for the money it spends? Said slightly differently, does the United States get corresponding value from the money it spends on health care? The available data often do not provide clear answers. For example, among OECD countries in 2004, the United States had shorter-than-average life expectancy and higher-than-average mortality rates. Does this mean that the U.S. system is inefficient in light of how much is spent on health care? Or does this reflect the greater prevalence of certain diseases in the United States (the United States has the highest incidence of cancer and AIDS in the OECD) and less healthy lifestyles (the United States has the highest obesity rates in the OECD)? These are some of the issues that confound international comparisons.

However, research comparing the quality of care has not found the United States to be superior overall. Nor does the U.S. population have substantially better access to health care resources, even putting aside the issue of the uninsured. Although the United States does not have long wait times for non-emergency surgeries, unlike some OECD countries, Americans found it more difficult to make same-day doctor's appointments when sick and had the most difficulty getting care on nights and weekends. They were also most likely to delay or forgo treatment because of cost.

The OECD data and other research provide some insight as to why health care spending is higher in the United States than in other countries, although many difficult research issues remain. This book presents some of the available data and research and concludes with a summary of study findings.

Chapter 1

HOW MUCH DOES THE UNITED STATES SPEND ON HEALTH CARE?[*]

ABSTRACT

The United States spends more money on health care than any other country in the Organization for Economic Cooperation and Development (OECD). The OECD consists of 30 democracies, most of which are considered the most economically advanced countries in the world. According to OECD data, the United States spent $6,102 per capita on health care in 2004 — more than double the OECD average and 19.9% more than Luxembourg, the second-highest spending country. In 2004, 15.3% of the U.S. economy was devoted to health care, compared with 8.9% in the average OECD country and 11.6% in second-placed Switzerland.

Why does the United States spend this amount on health care? Economists break health care spending into two parts: price and quantity (which includes the number of visits to health care providers and the intensity of those visits). In terms of quantity, OECD data indicate that the United States has far fewer doctor visits per person compared with the OECD average; for hospitalizations, the United States ranks well below the OECD and is roughly comparable in terms of length of hospital stays. The intensity of service delivery is a different story: the United States uses more of the newest medical technologies and performs several invasive procedures (such as coronary bypasses and angioplasties) more frequently than the

---

[*] Excerpted from CRS Report RL34715 dated September 17, 2007

average OECD country. In terms of price, the OECD has stated that "there is no doubt that U.S. prices for medical care commodities and services are significantly higher than in other countries and serve as a key determinant of higher overall spending."

What does the United States get for the money it spends? Said slightly differently, does the United States get corresponding value from the money it spends on health care? The available data often do not provide clear answers. For example, among OECD countries in 2004, the United States had shorter-than-average life expectancy and higher-than-average mortality rates. Does this mean that the U.S. system is inefficient in light of how much is spent on health care? Or does this reflect the greater prevalence of certain diseases in the United States (the United States has the highest incidence of cancer and AIDS in the OECD) and less healthy lifestyles (the United States has the highest obesity rates in the OECD)? These are some of the issues that confound international comparisons.

However, research comparing the quality of care has not found the United States to be superior overall. Nor does the U.S. population have substantially better access to health care resources, even putting aside the issue of the uninsured. Although the United States does not have long wait times for non-emergency surgeries, unlike some OECD countries, Americans found it more difficult to make same-day doctor's appointments when sick and had the most difficulty getting care on nights and weekends. They were also most likely to delay or forgo treatment because of cost.

The OECD data and other research provide some insight as to why health care spending is higher in the United States than in other countries, although many difficult research issues remain. This book presents some of the available data and research and concludes with a summary of study findings.

In 2004, health care spending in the United States averaged $6,102 per person, according to data from the Organization for Economic Cooperation and Development (OECD). The OECD consists of 30 democracies (listed in table 1), most of which are considered to be the most economically advanced countries in the world.[1]

As shown in figure 1 and table 1, U.S. per capita health care spending was well over double the average of OECD countries, which was $2,560 in 2004. Health care made up 15.3% of the U.S. economy in 2004, as measured by Gross Domestic Product (GDP) — up from 5.1% of GDP in 1960. No other OECD country devotes as much of its economy to health care, also shown in table 1.

Figure 2 shows the relationship between health care spending and GDP. The trendline in the figure suggests, based on a simple bivariate comparison, that 90% of the variation in health care spending across the 30 OECD countries may be attributable to GDP per capita. The two outliers are Luxembourg and the United

States. Luxembourg appears below the trendline because of its high GDP per capita, which is inflated by its international financial services.[2] The United States appears above the trendline because of its high health care spending; specifically, U.S. health care spending per capita is 60% higher than might be expected, based on GDP. U.S. health care spending is high, even when taking into account how rich the country is.

The next section of this book examines the volume, intensity, and price of U.S. health care and assesses the potential impact of each on U.S. spending. The following section discusses some structural causes affecting health care spending, such as the underlying health of countries' populations, which may be partially linked to demographics. Although such structural factors can affect health care spending substantially, quantifying that impact for international comparisons is difficult.

Finally, this book looks into the questions of what the United States gets for its health care spending and whether it spends "too much."

Table 1. Health Care Spending in OECD Countries, 2004

Country	Health care spending per capita	Health care spending per capita, as a percentage of U.S. amount	Health care spending as a percentage of GDP	GDP per capita	Percentage of health care publicly financed
United States	$6,102	100.0%	15.3%	$39,772	44.7%
Luxembourg	$5,089	83.4%	8.0%	$63,453	90.4%
Switzerland	$4,077	66.8%	11.6%	$35,149	58.4%
Norway	$3,966	65.0%	9.7%	$40,715	83.5%
Iceland	$3,331	54.6%	10.2%	$32,527	83.4%
Canada	$3,165	51.9%	9.9%	$31,828	69.8%
France	$3,159	51.8%	10.5%	$29,945	78.4%
Austria	$3,124	51.2%	9.6%	$32,519	70.7%
Australia	$3,120	51.1%	9.6%	$32,573	67.5%
Belgium	$3,044	49.9%	10.1%	$31,381	71.1%
Germany	$3,043	49.9%	10.6%	$28,816	76.9%
Netherlands	$3,041	49.8%	9.2%	$32,978	62.3%
Denmark	$2,881	47.2%	8.9%	$32,304	82.9%
Sweden	$2,825	46.3%	9.1%	$31,139	84.9%
Ireland	$2,596	42.5%	7.1%	$36,479	79.5%
United Kingdom	$2,508	41.1%	8.1%	$30,822	86.3%
Italy	$2,467	40.4%	8.7%	$28,352	75.1%
Japan	$2,249	36.9%	8.0%	$29,567	81.5%
Finland	$2,235	36.6%	7.5%	$29,778	76.6%
Greece	$2,162	35.4%	10.0%	$21,586	52.8%
Spain	$2,094	34.3%	8.1%	$25,875	70.9%
New Zealand	$2,083	34.1%	8.4%	$24,744	77.4%
Portugal	$1,824	29.9%	10.1%	$18,125	73.2%
Czech Republic	$1,361	22.3%	7.3%	$18,634	89.2%
Hungary	$1,276	20.9%	8.0%	$15,948	71.9%

Table 1. (Continued).

Country	Health care spending per capita	Health care spending per capita, as a percentage of U.S. amount	Health care spending as a percentage of GDP	GDP per capita	Percentage of health care publicly financed
Korea	$1,149	18.8%	5.6%	$20,668	51.4%
Poland	$805	13.2%	6.5%	$12,409	68.6%
Slovak Republic	$777	12.7%	5.9%	$14,060	88.3%
Mexico	$662	10.8%	6.5%	$10,242	46.4%
Turkey	$580	9.5%	7.7%	$7,562	72.1%
AVERAGE	$2,560	42.0%	8.9%	$27,998	72.9%
excluding U.S.	$2,438	39.9%	8.6%	$27,592	73.8%
Median	$2,552	41.8%	8.8%	$29,862	74.2%

Source: OECD Health Data 2006 (October 2006), with Congressional Research Service calculations.

Notes: GDP is Gross Domestic Product. Dollars are adjusted using U.S. dollar purchasing power parities, which convert currency from different countries into a common U.S. currency and equalize the purchasing power of different currencies. Health care spending per capita and spending as a percentage of GDP are based on estimates or prior-year spending for 15 countries (Belgium, Canada, Czech Republic, Denmark, France, Greece, Iceland, Japan, Luxembourg, Netherlands, Portugal, Slovak Republic, Spain, Sweden, and Switzerland). Data on the percentage of health care publicly financed in Denmark is from 2002. More information on the sources and methodology of country-specific health expenditure and finance data is available online at [http://www.irdes.fr/ecosante/OCDE/ 500.html].

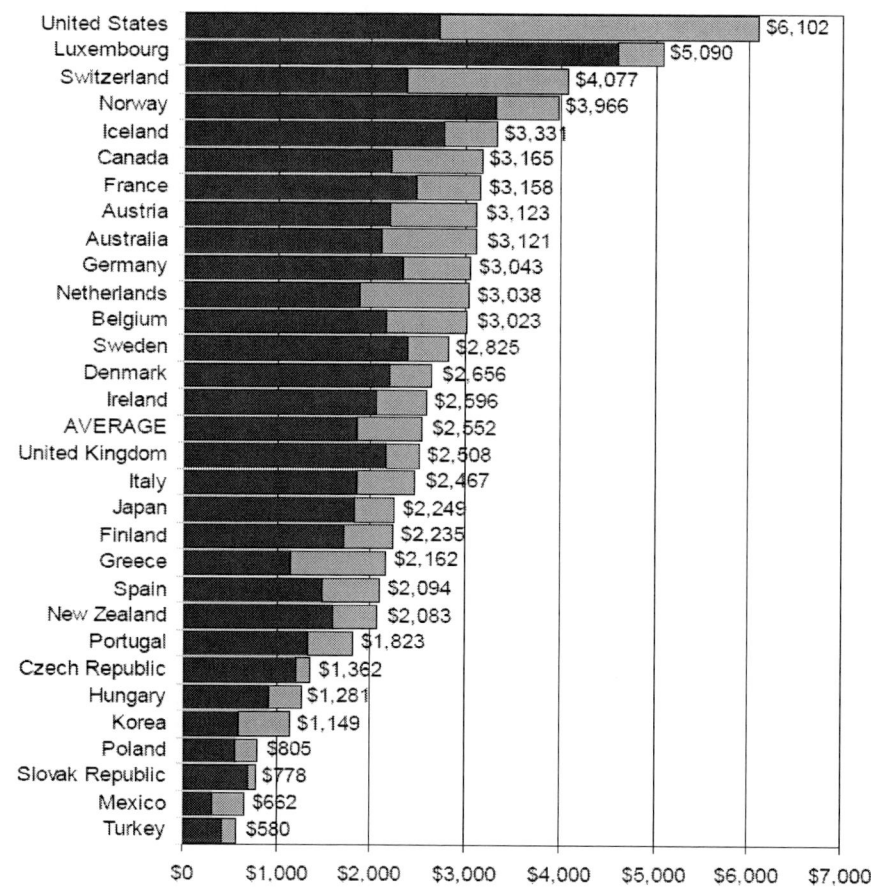

Source: OECD Health Data 2006 (October 2006).

Notes: Average per capita spending does not exactly match the amount in table 1 due to the use of data from different years for a few countries and other methodological issues. Dollars are adjusted using U.S. dollar purchasing power parities. Health care spending is based on estimates or on a previous year's spending for 15 countries: for Canada, the Czech Republic, France, Greece, Iceland, Luxembourg, the Netherlands, Portugal, Spain, Sweden, and Switzerland, the numbers are 2004 estimates; for Belgium, Japan, and the Slovak Republic, the numbers are from 2003; and for Denmark, the numbers are from 2002. More information on the sources and methodology of country-specific health expenditure and finance data is available online [http://www.irdes.fr/ecosante/OCDE/500.html].

Figure 1. Health Care Spending per Capita, 2004.

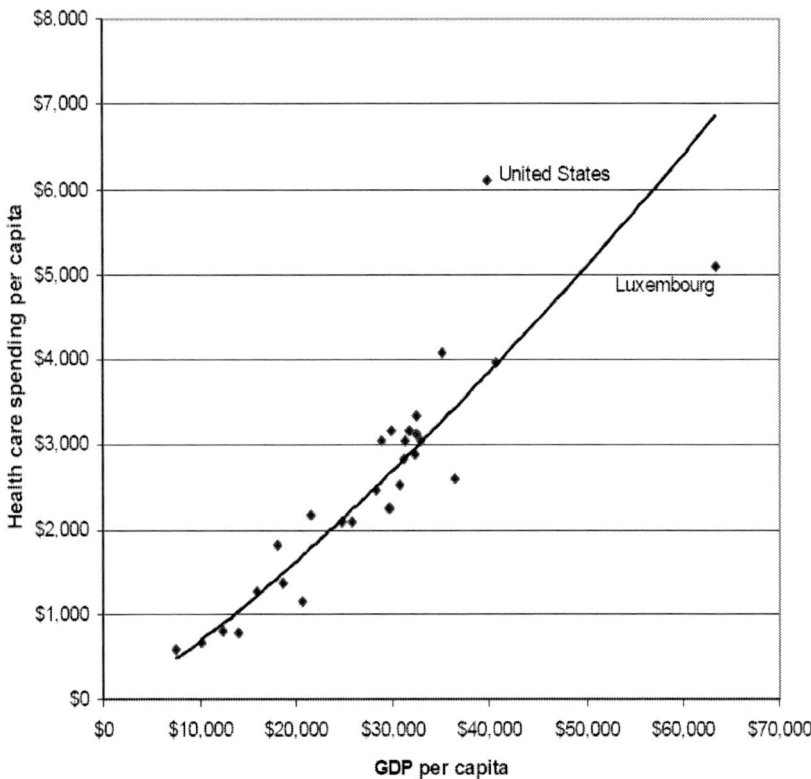

Source: Congressional Research Service (CRS) analysis of OECD Health Data 2006 (October 2006).

Notes: Health care spending is based on estimates or on prior-year spending for Belgium, Canada, Czech Republic, Denmark, France, Greece, Iceland, Japan, Luxembourg, Netherlands, Portugal, Slovak Republic, Spain, Sweden and Switzerland). More information on the sources of country specific expenditure and finance data is available online [http://www.irdes.fr/ecosante/ OCDE/500.html]. GDP is Gross Domestic Product. The R-squared for this trendline is 0.90.

Figure 2. Health Care Spending per Capita and GDP per Capita, 2004.

Chapter 2

WHY DOES THE UNITED STATES SPEND SO MUCH ON HEALTH CARE?

The standard economic approach to analyzing health care spending is to break it into two parts — price and quantity — because spending is calculated by multiplying the volume of units purchased by the unit price. However, health care spending is more complicated because for a particular "unit" (e.g., a hospital admission or a doctor visit), total spending will vary by the intensity of care. For example, two hospitals may charge the same price for particular services. Following a heart attack, when individuals are admitted to the hospitals, total spending is going to vary according to the intensity of care — whether patients undergo expensive surgeries or are simply given certain medications and monitored. To understand U.S. health care spending in an international context, this section examines the volume (or utilization) of certain types of health care, the intensity of care, and the price of care.

Chapter 3

VOLUME: DO AMERICANS USE HEALTH CARE MORE OFTEN?

When comparing U.S. utilization of hospital care with other OECD countries, the United States is well below the average. As shown in figure 3, the United States experienced 121 hospital discharges per 1,000 people in 2004, compared with the OECD average of 161. One possible explanation for the low U.S. utilization of hospital care is that services that are available in outpatient settings in the United States are available only in inpatient hospital settings in some European countries.

Diseases of the circulatory system were the largest single cause of hospitalizations in the OECD, accounting for 13% of all discharges. The United States had the highest proportion of hospital discharges because of diseases of the circulatory system (17%). Although the U.S. *proportion* was the highest in the OECD, the U.S. *number* of hospitalizations for circulatory-system diseases per 1,000 people in the population (21 per 1,000 people) was the same as the OECD average (as shown in the right-hand portion of figure 3). This is because of the low U.S. hospitalization utilization generally.

In 2004, physician services made up 22% of U.S. health care spending, second only to hospital care. When comparing per capita doctor visits in 27 OECD countries, the United States is the seventh lowest consumer of doctor visits, as shown in figure 4.[3] Among the four countries with the highest overall spending after the United States — Luxembourg, Switzerland, Norway and Iceland — their average number of doctor visits was also below the OECD average. Countries with higher rates of doctor visits tended to have lower overall health spending. The number of doctor visits per capita may be influenced by whether patients are required to get a referral in order to see a specialist; in the United States, such "gatekeeping," has subsided in recent years, whereas some European countries rely on this practice a great deal.

The next-largest component of health care spending in the United States in 2004 was prescription drugs. According to the OECD data, the United States spent roughly twice as much on prescription drugs ($752 per person) as the average OECD country in 2004 (figure 18). But because overall health spending per capita is even higher than in the average OECD country, prescription drugs ended up comprising a smaller portion of total U.S. health spending (12.3%) compared with the OECD average (17.8%) (figure 19).

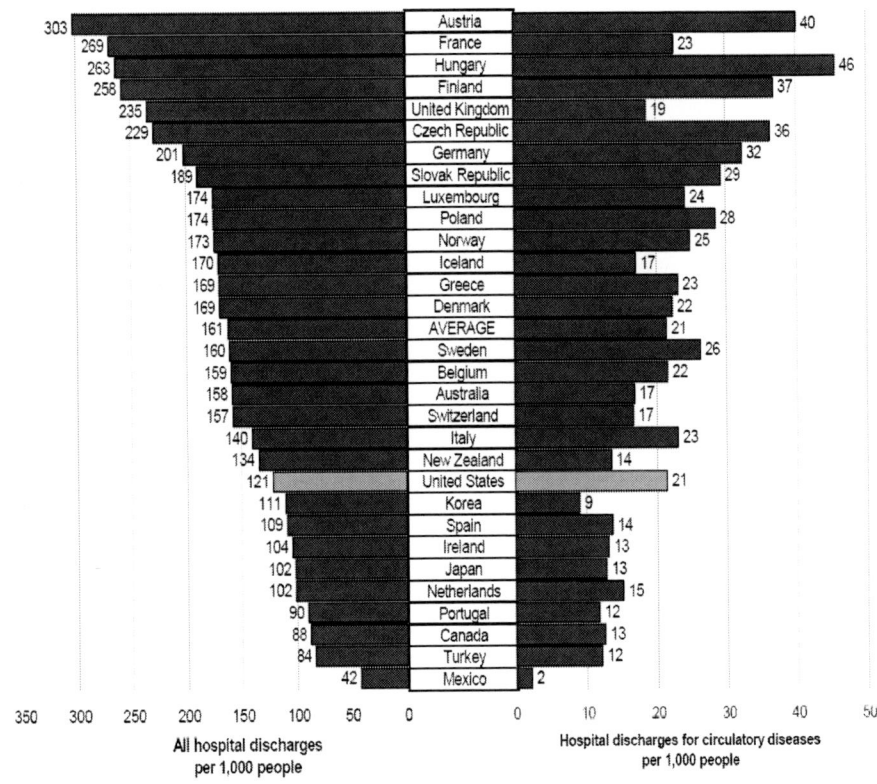

Source: OECD Health Data 2006 (October 2006).

Notes: Sorted by hospital utilization for all causes. Circulatory conditions include acute myocardial infarction (heart attack), angina pectoris, hypertensive diseases, and cerebrovascular diseases affecting blood flow to the brain. Data are from a previous year for 11 countries: for Belgium, Canada, Denmark, Germany, Italy, Mexico, Spain, and the United States, the data are from 2003; for Japan and Korea, the data are from 2002; and for Greece, the data are from 2000.

Figure 3. Hospital Utilization, for All Causes and for Circulatory Conditions, 2004.

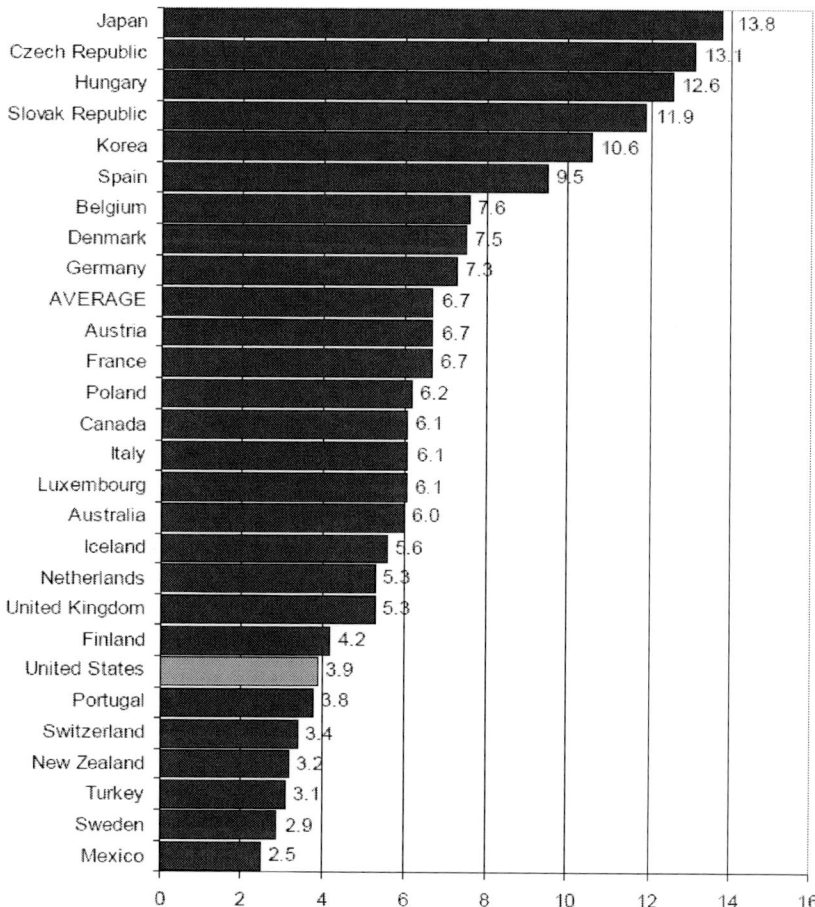

Source: OECD Health Data 2006 (October 2006).

Notes: The OECD defines doctor visits per capita as ambulatory contacts with physicians (both generalists and specialists) divided by the entire population. The number of contacts normally includes visits by patients to physicians' offices, primary care clinics, outpatient departments of hospitals, and visits made by a physician to a patient's home. Numbers are from a previous year for 12 countries: for Japan, Spain, France, Canada, the United States, and New Zealand, the data are from 2003; for Korea and Switzerland, the data are from 2002; for Iceland and Sweden, the data are from 2001; and for Germany and Italy, the data are from 2000. Recent data are only available for 27 of the 30 OECD countries. Greece, Ireland and Norway are not included.

Figure 4. Doctor Visits per Capita, 2004.

Chapter 4

INTENSITY: WHEN AMERICANS RECEIVE CARE, IS IT MORE INVOLVED?

The intensity of health care refers to the amount of resources used in a given health care encounter. For example, when similarly situated people are admitted to the hospital for a given condition, how many days do they remain in the hospital? How many tests do they undergo? Are the ancillary services costly? Do they require highly trained personnel? Do patients undergo surgery? Are those surgeries resource-intensive? Even when facilities charge the same price for services, the quantity of services provided during a health care encounter can have a huge impact on total spending.

Quantifying and comparing the intensity of health care, particularly across countries, is not simple. Ideally, one would compare the intensity of care (1) for similarly situated people, (2) for each type of health care event, and (3) according to the cause of the event. Some countries have a much older population that may require more intense care. Countries may also vary in terms of the prevalence of certain diseases in their populations. Moreover, intensity should be assessed by differentiating the cause of the health care event. For example, two similarly situated women may be admitted to a hospital, but if one is coming for normal childbirth and the other is coming for a heart transplant, the intensity of that hospital visit will be quite different. In the absence of such detailed data, the available aggregate measures (though less than ideal) are generally used.

Chapter 5

INTENSITY OF HOSPITALIZATIONS

One indicator of intensity is average length of acute care hospital stay, shown in figure 5.[4] Such a measure does not control for how the populations vary, nor for the causes of those hospitalizations. Some analysts prefer to use this measure as an indicator of efficiency — that shorter stays mean less health care spending. However, the services provided in those shorter stays could be much more intense compared with places where length of stays are longer. Thus, length of stay is far from an ideal measure of either intensity or efficiency. Moreover, if hospital stays are too short (that is, if sufficient inpatient treatment was not provided), then adverse health outcomes may result, along with potentially more health care spending. In 2004, the average length of a hospital stay in the United States was the same as the OECD average of 5.6 days.

Figure 6 shows the average length of stay following a heart attack (acute myocardial infarction). The United States average, 5.5 days, was the lowest in the OECD. Figure 7 shows the average length of stay for normal childbirth delivery. The United States had the third-lowest rate, 1.9 days — much shorter than the OECD average of 3.6 days.[5] In the absence of information about the price or quantity of the services provided during hospital stays, the lower than average hospital utilization and lengths of stay would suggest lower than average spending, which is not the case.

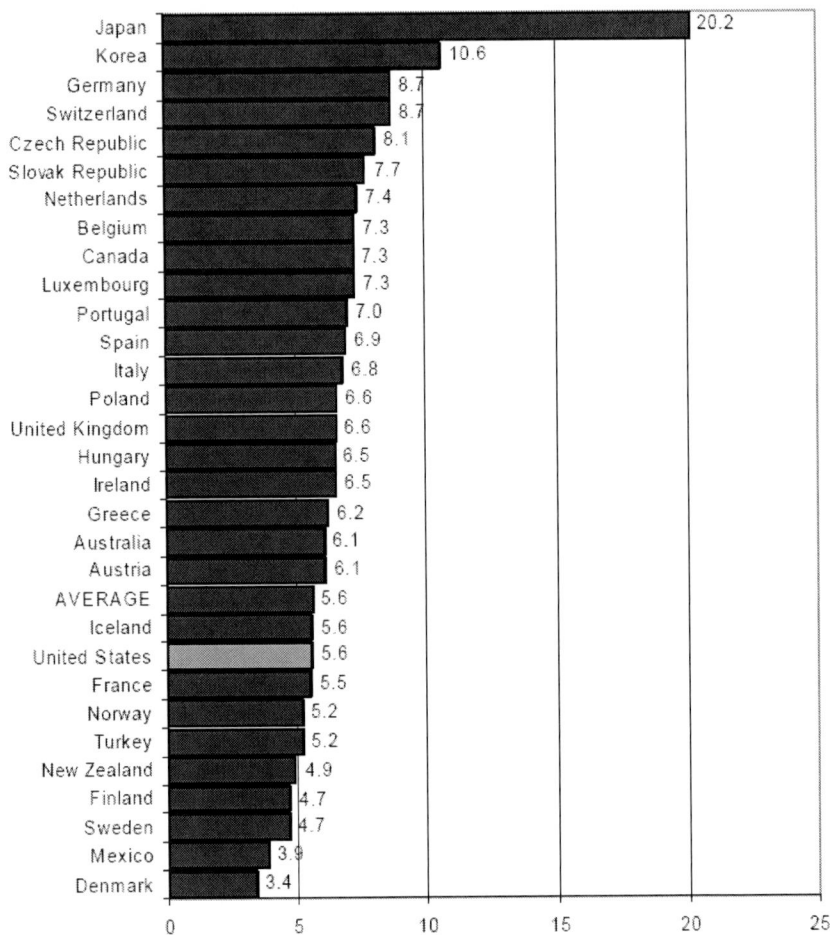

Source: OECD Health Data 2006 (October 2006).

Notes: Acute care is curative care generally provided in a hospital (as opposed to long-term care, which is generally provided in a nursing home). Numbers are from previous years for 10 countries: for Belgium, Italy, Korea, Mexico, Portugal, and Spain, the numbers are from 2003; for Turkey, the numbers are from 2002; for the Netherlands, the numbers are from 2001; for Greece, the numbers are from 2000; and for New Zealand, the numbers are from 1998. In Japan, most elderly patients requiring long-term care receive it in hospitals instead of nursing homes.[6]

Figure 5. Average Length of Acute Care Hospital Stay, Number of Days, 2004.

Intensity of Hospitalizations 17

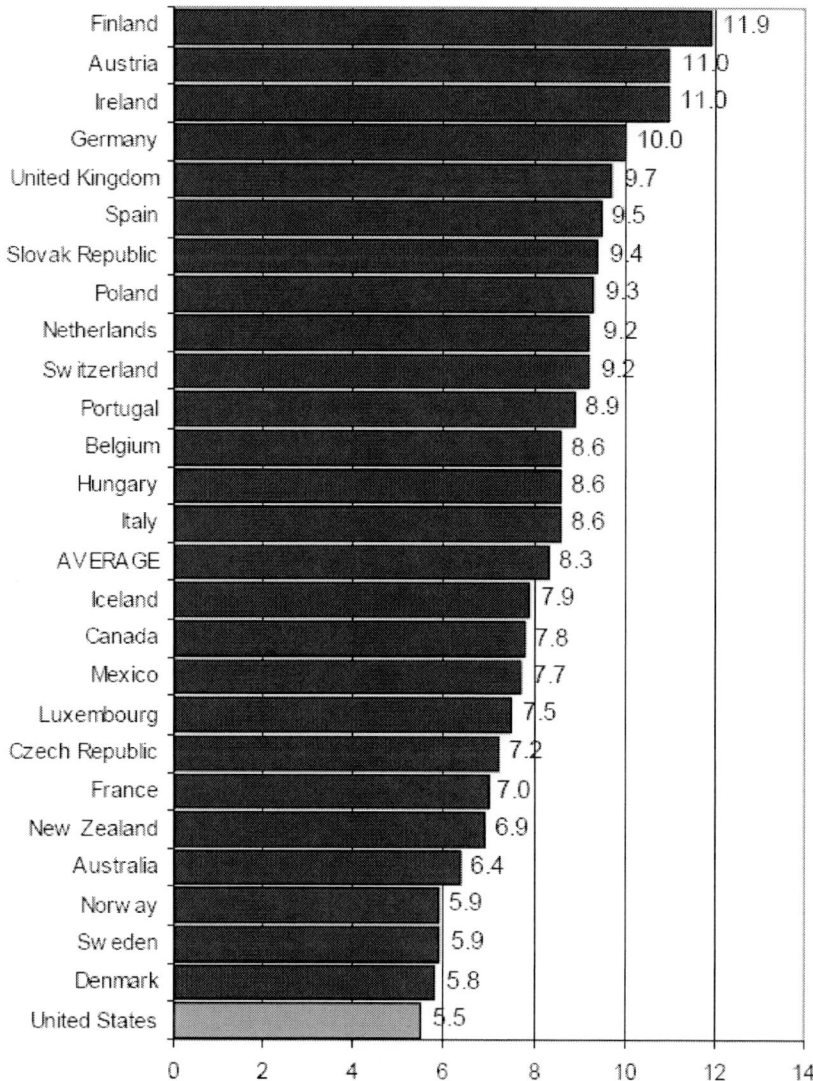

Source: OECD Health Data 2006 (October 2006).
Notes: Data from 2003 are available for only 26 of the 30 OECD countries.

Figure 6. Average Length of Hospital Stay Following Heart Attack, 2003.

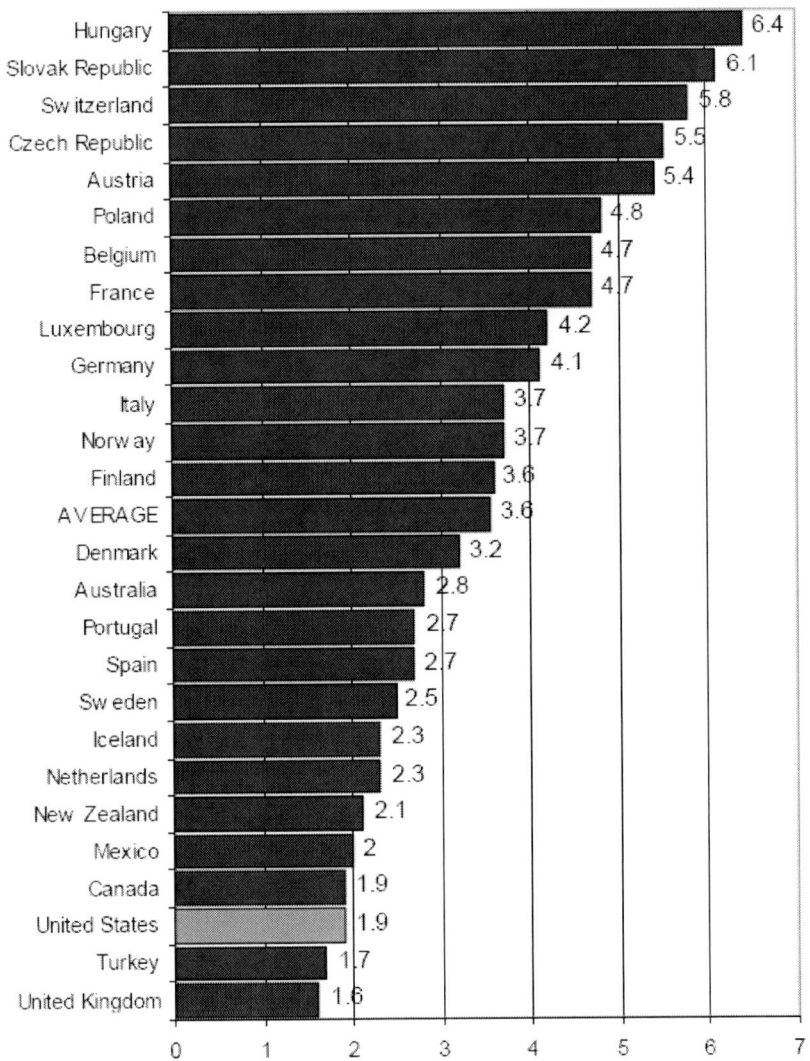

Source: OECD Health Data 2006 (October 2006).
Notes: Data from 2003 are available for only 26 of the 30 OECD countries.

Figure 7. Average Length of Hospital Stay Following Normal Childbirth, 2003.

Although U.S. hospital stays are generally fewer and shorter, the services provided during those stays may be particularly intensive. Some evidence suggests this is the case. Figure 8 shows that the United States has the fifth-highest rate of caesarean section childbirths. In addition, the United States has one of the top five highest rates of performing organ transplants — another particularly intensive type of procedure — for all but one type of organ.[7]

For all four types of heart procedures on which the OECD collects data, the United States consistently has one of the top five highest rates of performing such procedures. Figures 9 illustrates the use of two intensive surgical coronary revascularization procedures — coronary artery bypass grafts (CABGs) and coronary angioplasties (PTCAs). In 2003, these procedures were performed on 587 out of 100,000 people in the United States — more than double the OECD average.

That said, cross-national comparisons do not always indicate consistently high levels of U.S. service intensity. The United States ranks 2nd in its rate of knee replacements but 15th in its rate of hip replacements. The United States performed more procedures than the OECD median for six conditions in 2003, but *fewer* procedures than the OECD median for four other conditions.[8]

For acute care hospitalizations, other broad measures of intensity are the number of staff and the number of nurses per hospital bed. In 2003, the United States averaged five staff members for each occupied acute care hospital bed. This is 61% greater than the OECD average and second only to the United Kingdom (6.5 staff per bed), as shown in figure 10.[9] When looking at the rate of *nurses* per occupied bed, the United States is closer to the OECD average, as shown in figure 11.

Although the intensity of hospitalizations in the United States (measured by number of staff per bed and number of intensive procedures performed) tends to be above the OECD average, it rarely ranks first. The exceptions are coronary revascularization procedures and kidney transplants. For the coronary procedures in particular, not only did the United States rank first, but the rates of these procedures were far greater than any other OECD country.

Other important measures of hospital care intensity are usage rates of resource-intensive technologies. International comparisons of the usage of technologies such as computerized tomography (CT) scanners and magnetic resonance imaging units (MRIs) are not available. However, the OECD data include information on the prevalence of these technologies, which may indicate their usage. The United States has nearly twice as many CT scanners (figure 12) and three times as many MRI machines (figure 13) per capita as the OECD average. In fact, the United States has the second-highest number of both CT scanners and MRI machines per population in the OECD, second only to Japan, where low reimbursement rates have driven the development and widespread adoption of inexpensive versions of these machines.[10]

Widespread use of advanced medical technology can contribute to higher health spending in a number of ways: through the cost of the equipment or machines themselves; by keeping people alive longer and thereby increasing the opportunity for them to use health care; through eventual expansions in the populations being treated with these technologies; and because competition between hospitals can lead to an oversupply of machines, which in turn can lead to increases in health spending.[11]

Chapter 6

INTENSITY OF DOCTOR VISITS

The number of doctor visits per capita in the United States was well below the OECD average in 2004 (figure 4), yet the United States spent much more per capita on outpatient care than any other OECD country. The United States spent $2,668 per capita on outpatient care alone in 2004 — three-and-a-half times the OECD average and twice as much as the second-highest spender in this category. As mentioned earlier, this discrepancy could be partially due to the tendency to provide more types of procedures in outpatient settings in the United States compared with many other OECD countries.

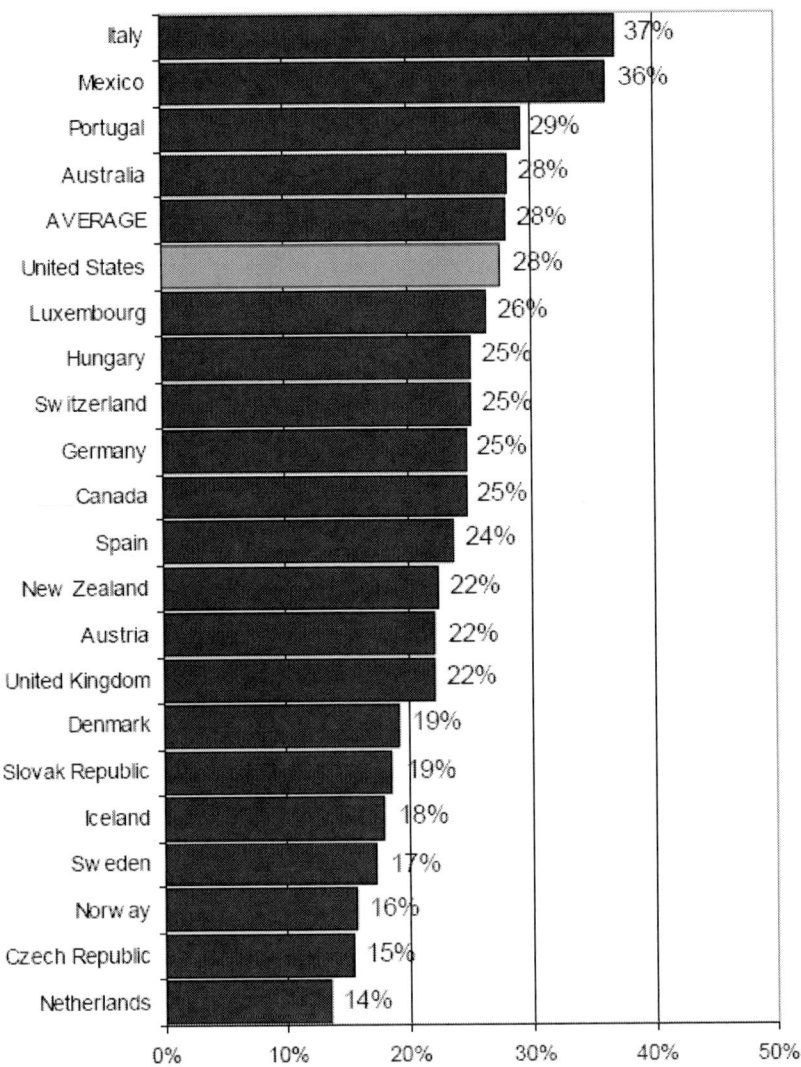

Source: OECD Health Data 2006 (October 2006).
Note: Coronary revascularization procedures are coronary artery bypass grafts (CABGs) and coronary angioplasties (PTCAs) and stenting. Caesarean section data from 2003 are available only for 21 of the 30 OECD countries. Coronary revascularization data from 2003 are available only for 19 of the 30 OECD countries. In figure 9, the median (207) is also shown because the average (332) is so skewed by the U.S. rate.

Figure 8. Percentage of Live Births that Are Caesarean Sections, 2003.

Intensity of Doctor Visits 23

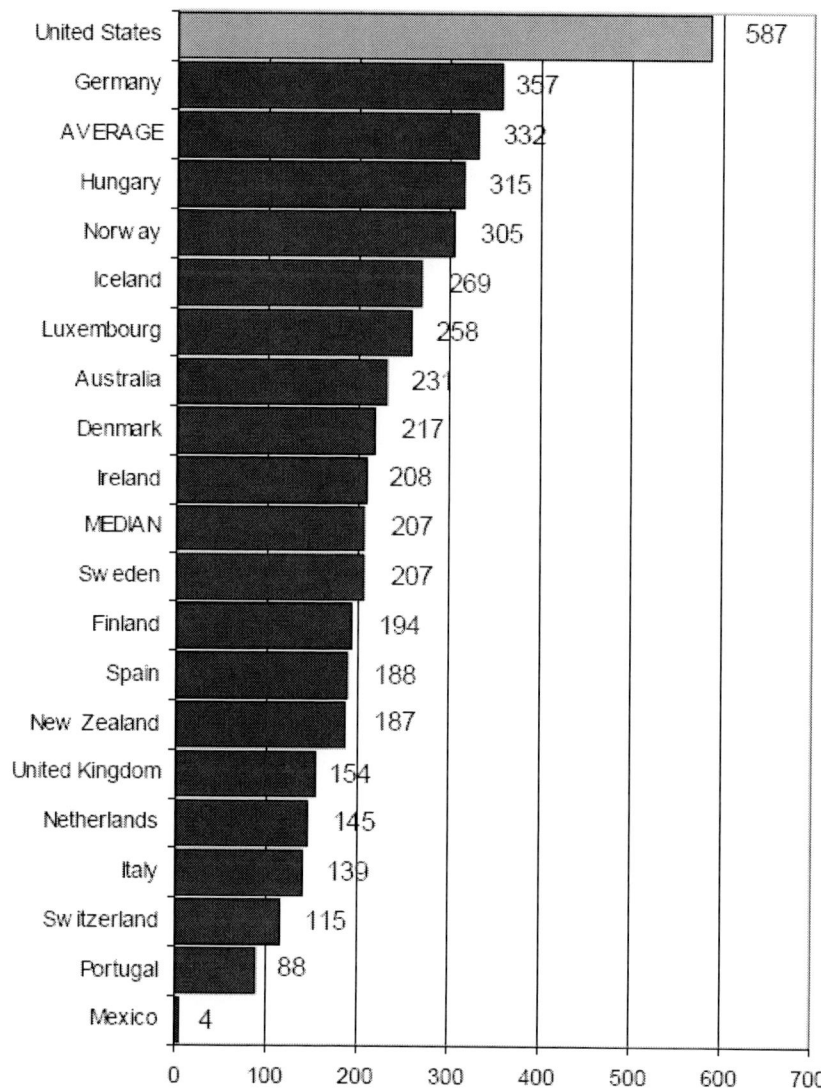

Source: OECD Health Data 2006 (October 2006).
Note: Coronary revascularization procedures are coronary artery bypass grafts (CABGs) and coronary angioplasties (PTCAs) and stenting. Caesarean section data from 2003 are available only for 21 of the 30 OECD countries. Coronary revascularization data from 2003 are available only for 19 of the 30 OECD countries. In figure 9, the median (207) is also shown because the average (332) is so skewed by the U.S. rate.

Figure 9. Rate (per 100,000 population) of Coronary Revascularization Procedures, 2003.

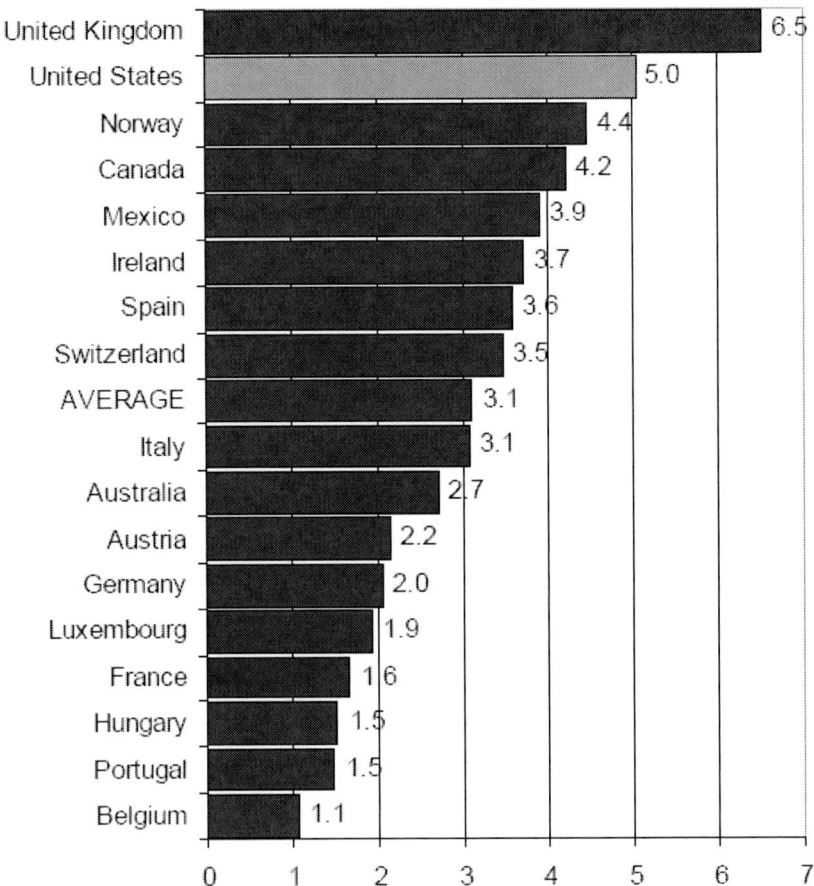

Source: CRS analysis of OECD Health Data 2006 (October 2006).

Notes: Numbers may not be directly comparable because some countries calculate using Full Time Equivalent staff, whereas others use headcounts. Data on staff per bed from 2003 are available for only 17 of the 30 OECD countries. Data on nurses per bed from 2003 are available for only 18 of the 30 OECD countries.

Figure 10. Number of Staff per Acute Care Hospital Bed, 2003.

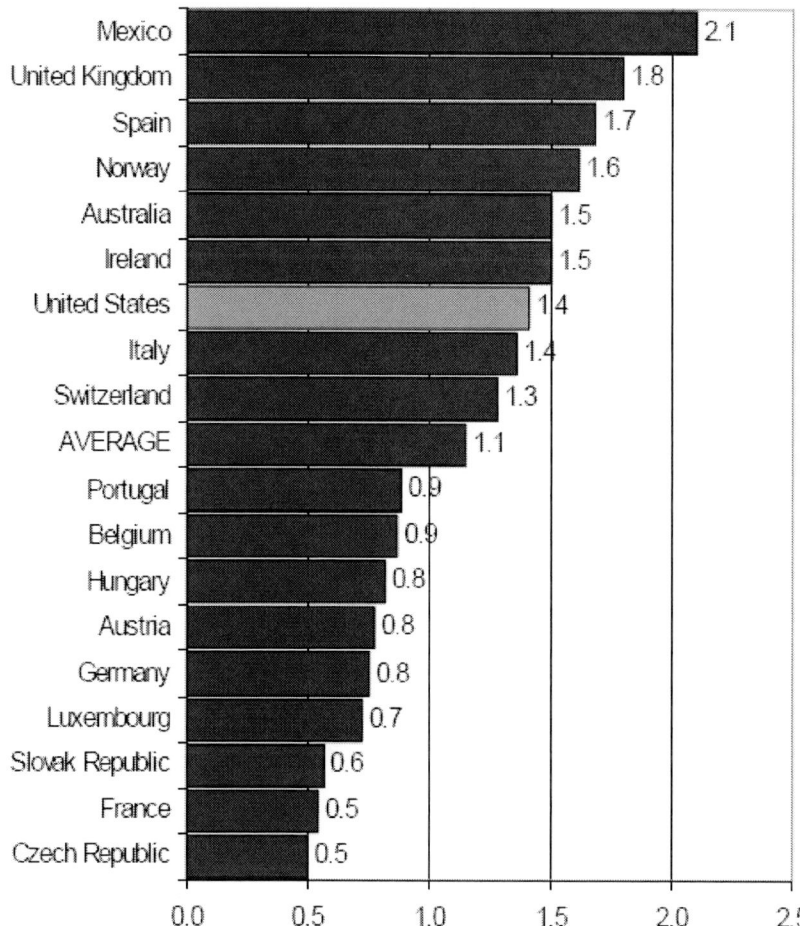

Source: CRS analysis of OECD Health Data 2006 (October 2006).
Notes: Numbers may not be directly comparable because some countries calculate using Full Time Equivalent staff, whereas others use headcounts. Data on staff per bed from 2003 are available for only 17 of the 30 OECD countries. Data on nurses per bed from 2003 are available for only 18 of the 30 OECD countries.

Figure 11. Number of Nurses per Acute Care Hospital Bed, 2003.

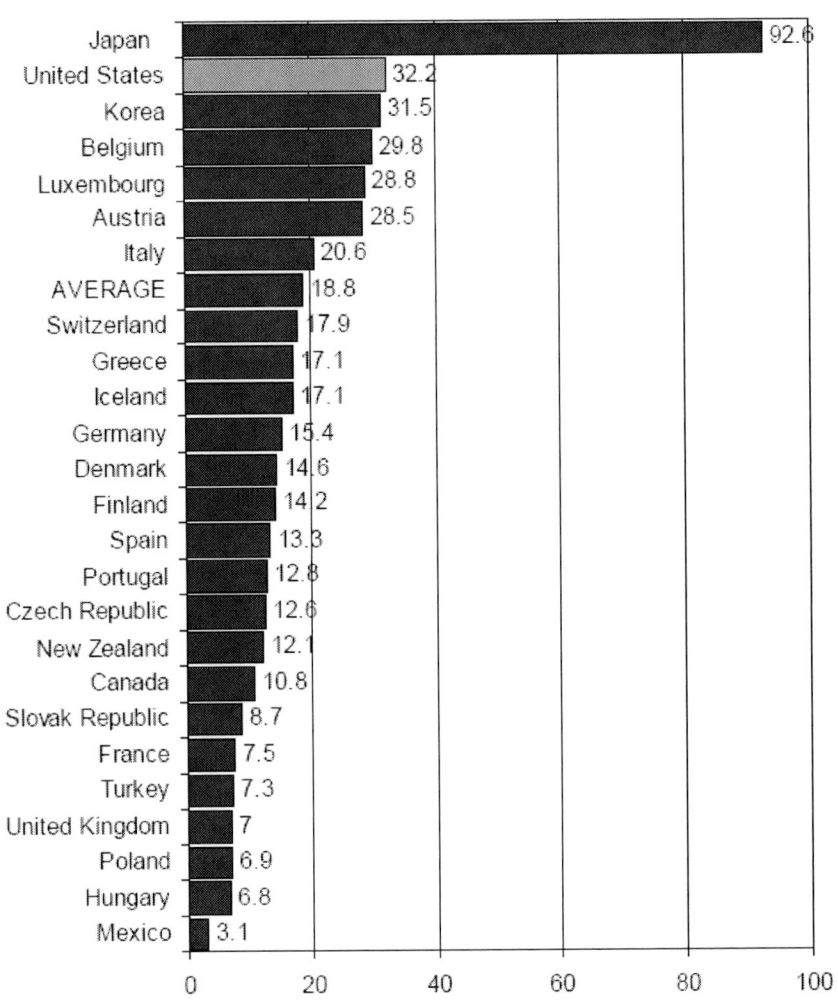

Source: OECD Health Data 2006 (October 2006).

Notes: Data for Belgium, Portugal, the Slovak Republic, and Turkey are from 2003; data for Greece and Japan are from 2002. Data on CT scanners from 2004 are available for only 25 of the 30 OECD countries.

Figure 12. Number of CT Scanners per 1,000,000 Population, 2004.

Intensity of Doctor Visits 27

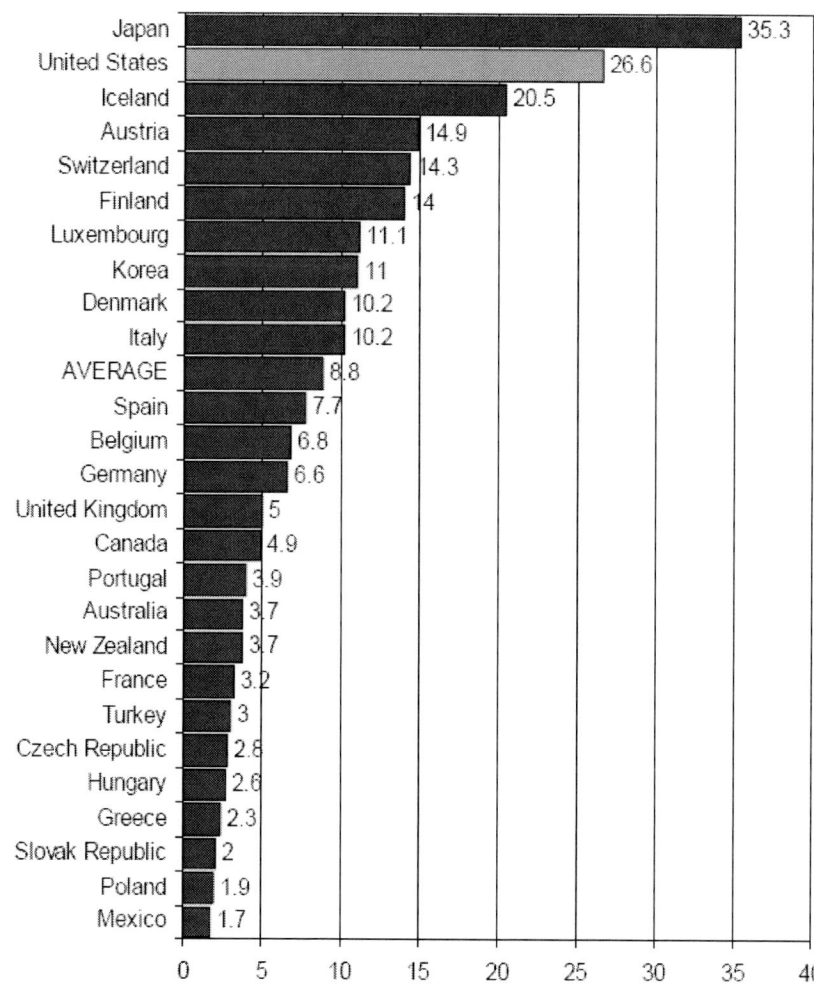

Source: OECD Health Data 2006 (October 2006).
Notes: Data for Belgium, New Zealand, Portugal, and the Slovak Republic are from 2003; data for Greece and Japan are from 2002. Data on MRI machines from 2004 are available for only 26 of the 30 OECD countries.

Figure 13. Number of MRI Units per 1,000,000 Population, 2004.

Chapter 7

INTRA-NATIONAL VARIATION IN INTENSITY

It is necessary to note that there is a major amount of variation in health care intensity *within* the United States. For example, research by John Wennberg and his colleagues at Dartmouth College found that "age-, sex-, and race-adjusted spending for traditional, fee-for-service (FFS) Medicare in the Miami hospital referral region in 1996 was $8,414 — nearly two and a half times the $3,341 spent that year in the Minneapolis region."[12] They ruled out utilization of surgical procedures and price as the main drivers of these differences. Instead, they concluded that "end-of-life care makes Miami truly exceptional: Patients in their last six months of life see more physicians and spend more time in intensive care than is the case virtually anywhere else."[13]

Thus, to the extent that one concludes that U.S. spending levels are the highest in the world because of the intensity of care, it should be noted that level of intensity is not nationwide and is not consistently high for all services and for all similarly situated individuals within the United States.

Chapter 8

PRICE: DO AMERICANS PAY MORE FOR HEALTH CARE SERVICES?

As previously discussed, Americans do not lead the world in per capita doctor visits or hospitalizations. When Americans receive health care services, they appear to receive a higher-than-average amount of certain surgical procedures and advanced medical technologies, but generally do not have the *highest* levels in the OECD. This leaves price as the last remaining factor in the equation to explain the high level of U.S. health care spending.

In assessing what drives the difference between U.S. health care spending and the rest of the world, some leading health economists responded this way: "It's the prices, stupid."[14] Put more formally, a report from the OECD declared that "there is no doubt that U.S. prices for medical care commodities and services are significantly higher than in other countries and serve as a key determinant of higher overall spending."[15]

While there is little disagreement that prices are a "key determinant" of higher U.S. health care spending, direct comparisons of international prices of health care goods and services are extremely difficult, requiring analysts to answer some vexing methodological questions. For example, what index, among the various exchange rates and purchasing power parities (PPPs), should be used for currency conversion? Price comparisons are quite sensitive to these assumptions. What are the units to be priced — for example, the average cost of an entire surgical procedure or the charges for components of the procedure (hourly rate of the health professionals, charges for equipment usage, etc.)? By choosing the former, intensity is inappropriately subsumed into the "price"; however, the latter is difficult to ascertain for all the components of the procedure. Certainly, such price information is rare in an aggregate form that is comparable across multiple countries.

This section of the report presents some price comparisons of certain health care goods and services. These comparisons are by no means exhaustive in covering the entire health care system, and require some of the methodological caveats alluded to earlier.

Chapter 9

SALARIES OF HEALTH PROFESSIONALS

Standard economic theory teaches that the production of any good or service requires labor and/or capital. Health care is particularly labor-intensive, requiring the involvement of many individuals, including numerous highly trained professionals such as doctors and nurses. Total health care costs, therefore, will partly be a function of the price of labor — doctors' and nurses' salaries, for instance. As it turns out, U.S. health care professionals (specialists, general practitioners, and nurses) are among the highest paid health professionals in the world. As shown in table 2, specialists are the third-highest paid, and general practitioners and nurses are the highest paid within their profession among reporting OECD countries.

It is necessary to note, however, that higher education in most of the OECD is much less expensive (or even free) compared with the United States. As a result, health care professionals in the rest of the OECD generally begin their careers with considerably smaller educational debts compared with those in the United States. In 2006, 86.7% of new medical school graduates had outstanding educational loans, with an average total educational debt of $129,943.[16] Depending on how the repayment is structured, the annual payments could be as low as $7,000 per year (with payments over 30 years) or as high as $18,000 per year (with payments over 10 years).

Table 2. Average Compensation in Certain Health Professions, 2004 (Dollars in U.S. Purchasing Power Parities)

	Specialists		General practitioners		Nurses	
	in $1,000s	Ratio to per capita GDP	in $1,000s	Ratio to per capita GDP	in $1,000s	Ratio to per capita GDP
Netherlands	$253	6.0	$117	3.6		
Australia	$247	7.6	$91	2.8	$48	1.5
United States	$230	5.7	$161	4.1	$56	1.4
Belgium	$188	6.0	$61	2.0		
Canada	$161	5.1	$107	3.4		
United Kingdom	$150	4.9	$118	3.9	$42	1.4
France	$149	5.0	$92	3.1		
Ireland	$143	4.0			$41	1.1
Switzerland	$130	3.8	$116	3.4		
Denmark	$91	2.9	$109	3.4	$42	1.3
New Zealand	$89	3.6			$34	1.4
Germany	$77	2.7				
Norway	$77	1.9			$35	0.9
Sweden	$76	2.5	$66	2.2		
Finland	$74	2.5	$68	2.3	$29	1.0
Greece	$67	3.1			$33	1.5
Portugal	$64	3.5	$64	3.5	$34	1.9
Czech Republic	$35	1.7	$32	1.7	$14	0.8
Hungary	$27	1.7	$26	1.6	$14	0.9
Mexico	$25	2.4	$21	2.1	$13	1.3
Poland	$20	1.6				
AVERAGE	$113	3.7	$83	2.9	$33	1.3
excluding U.S.	$107	3.6	$78	2.8	$32	1.3
Median	$83	3.3	$80	3.0	$34	1.3

Source: Congressional Research Service (CRS) analysis of *Remuneration of Health Professions*, OECD Health Data 2006 (October 2006), available at [http://www.ecosante.fr/OCDEENG/70.html].

Notes: Sorted by specialists' compensation. Amounts are adjusted using U.S. dollar purchasing power parities. Amounts from previous years are trended up to 2004 dollars using the annualized Bureau of Labor Statistics Employment Cost Index for wages and salaries of health services workers in private industry. It is not known whether wage growth in health professions in other countries was similar to that in the United States. Amounts are from previous years for 10 countries: data for Australia, Canada, Denmark (for specialists and nurses), Finland (for nurses), and the Netherlands are from 2003; data for Belgium (for specialists), Denmark (for general practitioners), New Zealand (for nurses), and Sweden are from 2002; data for Switzerland and the United States (for specialists and general practitioners) are from

2001; and data for Belgium (for general practitioners) and the United States (for nurses) are from 2000. Ratios of salaries to GDP per capita reflect the year the data was collected and are not adjusted for inflation. For countries that have both self-employed and salaried professionals in a given field, the amount presented here is the higher of the two salaries. Four countries have both salaried and self-employed specialists: the Czech Republic (where compensation is $29,484 for salaried and $34,852 for self-employed specialists), Greece ($67,119 and $64,782), the Netherlands ($130,911 and $252,727), and the United States ($170,300 and $229,500). One country has both salaried and self-employed general practitioners: in the United States, salaried general practitioners earn $134,600, compared with $154,200 if self-employed. All nurses are salaried among this data. Recent data are available only for 21 of the 30 OECD countries.

Health professionals tend to be paid more generous salaries as the wealth of a country increases (indicated in table 2 by larger ratios of provider salaries to per capita GDP). Even accounting for this trend, however, the United States pays health professionals more than would be predicted by U.S. wealth. As an example, figure 14 presents specialist salaries and GDP per capita, with data points above the trendline indicating countries where salaries are more generous than GDP per capita would predict. The U.S. position above the trendline indicates that specialists are paid approximately $50,000 more than would be predicted by the high U.S. GDP. General practitioners are paid roughly $30,000 more than the U.S. GDP would predict, and nurses are paid $8,000 more (not shown).

In the labor market, salaries are typically determined by the supply of available workers. When relatively low numbers of professionals with appropriate training exist, they are able to command higher salaries, based on the scarcity of their skills. Figure 15 shows that the United States has a relatively low supply of practicing physicians, which could help explain their high salaries.

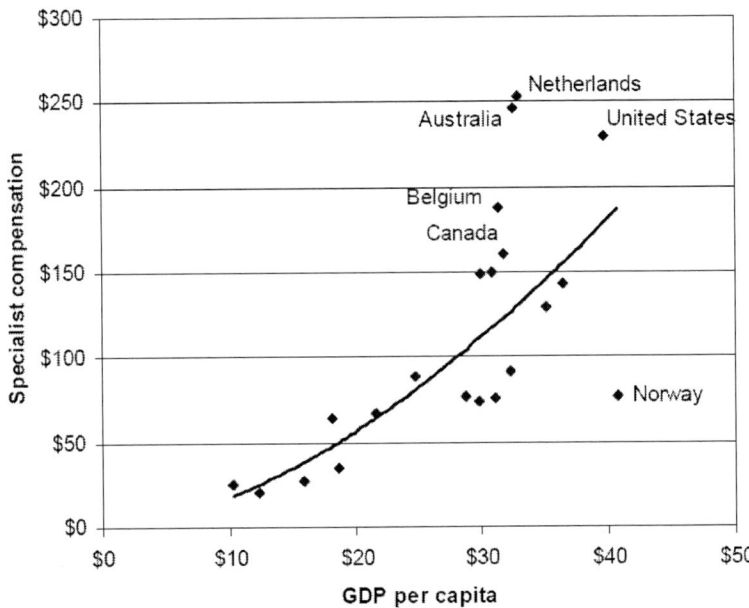

Source: Congressional Research Service (CRS) analysis of Remuneration of Health Professions, OECD Health Data 2006 (October 2006), available at [http://www.ecosante.fr/OCDEENG/70.html].

Notes: Amounts are adjusted using U.S. dollar purchasing power parities. Amounts are from previous years for 10 countries: data for Australia, Canada, Denmark, and the Netherlands are from 2003; data for Belgium and Sweden are from 2002; data for Switzerland and the United States are from 2001. Amounts from previous years are trended up to 2004 dollars using the annualized Bureau of Labor Statistics Employment Cost Index for wages and salaries of health services workers in private industry. It is not known whether wage growth in health professions in other countries was similar to that in the United States. For countries that have both self-employed and salaried professionals in a given field, the amount presented here is the higher of the two salaries. Four countries have both salaried and self-employed specialists: the Czech Republic (where compensation is $29,484 for salaried and $34,852 for self-employed specialists), Greece ($67,119 and $64,782), the Netherlands ($130,911 and $252,727), and the United States ($170,300 and $229,500). One country has both salaried and self-employed general practitioners: in the U.S., salaried general practitioners earn $134,600, compared with $154,200 if self-employed. All nurses are salaried among this data. Recent data are available only for 21 of the 30 OECD countries. The R-squared for this trendline is 0.72.

Figure 14. Specialist Compensation and GDP per Capita (in U.S. $1,000s), 2004.

Salaries of Health Professionals 37

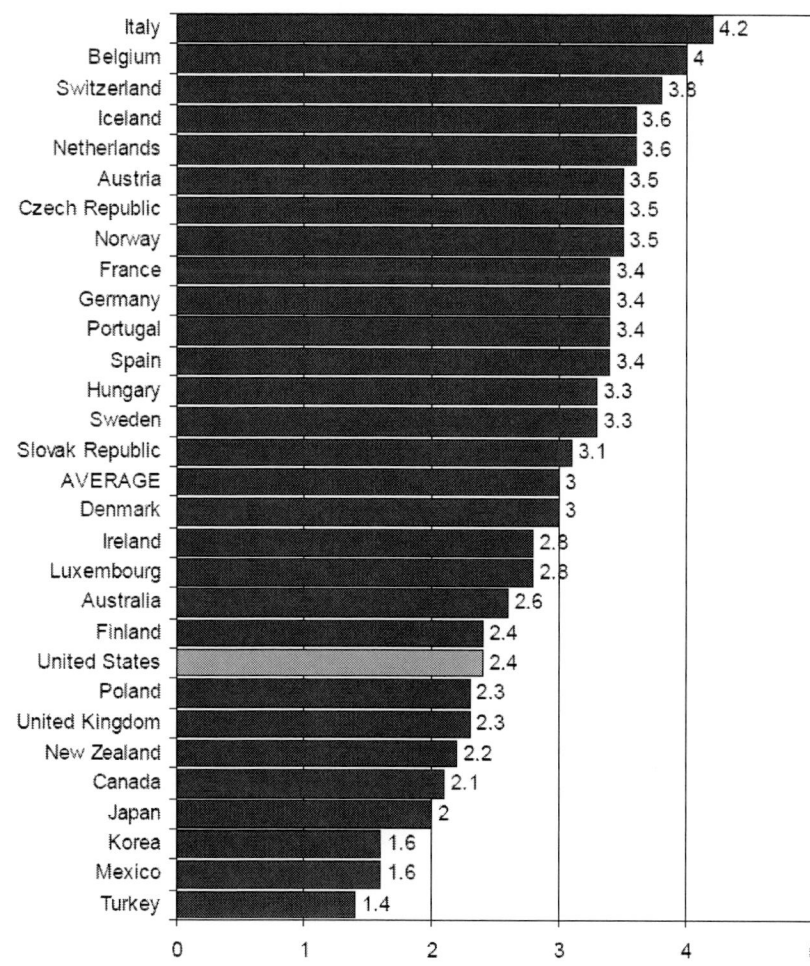

Source: OECD Health Data 2006 (October 2006).
Notes: Data for Australia, Denmark, New Zealand, Sweden, and Turkey are from 2003.
Recent data are available only for 29 of the 30 OECD countries.

Figure 15. Practicing Physicians per 1,000 Population, 2004.

Chapter 10

PRICE OF MEDICAL EQUIPMENT

Although it can be defined more broadly, capital in the classical economic sense generally refers to physical items used in the production of a good or service — a building, equipment, etc. For health care equipment in particular, it is widely believed that the United States pays the highest prices. Part of the cause may be that the United States is an early adopter of new technologies. The OECD data indicate that when CT scanners, MRIs, and lithotriptors were new technologies, the United States had more of these per capita than any other country. Higher introductory prices are paid by early adopters. However, OECD data comparing international prices of medical equipment, let alone other forms of health care capital, are not available.

Chapter 11

PRICE OF MEDICAL PROCEDURES

Although the OECD does not collect data comparing prices of medical procedures, several international studies have consistently found that the United States pays higher prices than other countries for medical procedures. One group of researchers compared in-hospital spending for total hip arthroplasty among patients in three teaching hospitals in Canada and three teaching hospitals in the United States over a five-year period. They found total spending for the procedure in the United States to be twice that in Canada — with both overhead costs and direct care costs twice the Canadian level, as shown in table 3. The spending on direct care in the United States was higher in spite of shorter hospital stays. Physician fees were not included in this analysis, but because they are generally much lower in Canada than in the United States, including that information would only increase the divergence in costs.[17]

Table 3. Average Spending for Treatment of Patients Who Had a Total Hip Arthroplasty

Spending	Canada	United States
Spending on direct care	$4,552 (67%)	$8,221 (62%)
Spending on overhead	$2,214 (33%)	$5,118 (38%)
Total spending	$6,766 (100%)	$13,339 (100%)

Source: Table II, John Antoniou et al., "In-Hospital Cost of Total Hip Arthroplasty in Canada and the United States," *Journal of Bone and Joint Surgery*, November 2004, vol. 86, no. 11, pp. 2435-2439.

Note: Reported spending in U.S. dollars. Canadian dollar spending amounts were converted to U.S. dollar amounts using purchasing power parities for 1997 through 2001.

The two other studies that have compared procedure prices in the United States and Canada have found similar results: coronary artery bypass graft surgery costs twice as much in the United States than in Canada,[18] and open abdominal aortic aneurysm repair costs 47% more in the United States than in Canada.[19]

Chapter 12

PRICE OF PHARMACEUTICALS

It is generally accepted that the United States pays higher prices for its prescription drugs than most of the world. How much more the United States pays continues to be debated. Direct international price comparisons of prescription drugs have been attempted over the years.

In the early 1990s, the Government Accountability Office (GAO) (then called the General Accounting Office) issued ground-breaking reports comparing U.S. prescription drug prices to those of Canada and the United Kingdom.[20] For the brand-name prescription drugs that were included in the GAO studies, the U.S. price averaged nearly 32% more than in Canada and 60% more than in the United Kingdom.[21] In spite of efforts to make valid comparisons, some other researchers argued that the U.S. numbers did not adequately reflect discounts and rebates given to HMOs, Medicaid, and other large purchasers.[22] In the intervening years, additional attempts have been made to perform international drug price comparisons, although many of the same limitations apply.

A 2003 study by Patricia M. Danzon and Michael F. Furukawa, compared drug prices in the United States with prices in eight other countries.[23] The drugs used in the study were the 249 leading molecules (active ingredients) in the United States. The study found that brand-name prescription drugs still under patent were most expensive in Japan, with the United States ranked second among the nine countries. In the other seven countries, on-patent prescription drug prices were 24% to 39% less expensive than in the United States, as shown in figure 16. However, among the generic drugs in the study, the United States had the second-*lowest* prices, also shown in figure 16.[24] For over-the-counter drugs, the United States had the lowest prices by far among the countries in the study. One commentator summarized the findings this way: "It is not accurate to say, then, that the United States has higher prescription-drug prices than other countries. It is accurate to say only that the United States has a different pricing system from that of other countries. Americans pay more for drugs when they first come out and less as the drugs get older, while the rest of the world pays less in the beginning and more later."[25]

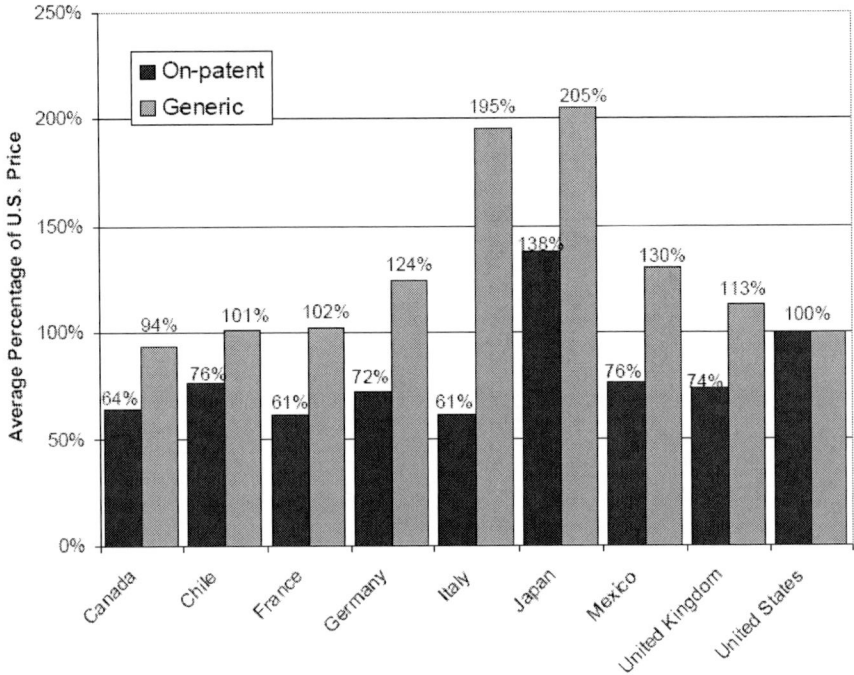

Source: Patricia M. Danzon and Michael F. Furukawa, "Prices and Availability of Pharmaceuticals: Evidence from Nine Countries," *Health Affairs*, Web exclusive, October 29, 2003, pp. W3-521-W3-536, available at [http://content.healthaffairs.org/cgi/reprint/hlthaff.w3.521v1.pdf], Exhibit 4; Patricia M. Danzon, "Drug Importation: Economic Impact," June 2004 presentation, available at [http://www.ehcca.com/presentations/pharmacolloquium1/danzon.pdf], slide 18.

Notes: "On-patent drugs" are brand-name prescription drugs available from only a single manufacturer that is also the company that developed the drug. The numbers represent the wholesale list prices (that is, the amount charged by manufacturers to wholesalers). The numbers also incorporate Danzon and Furukawa's estimates of "off-invoice discounts" in the United States, which reduced U.S. prices by approximately 8%. The comparisons are based on currency exchange rates rather than purchasing price parities (PPPs) because currency exchange rates will be the basis of manufacturers' decisions when projecting their sales revenue. Note that on-patent brand name drugs and off-patent generic drugs are not the same price in the United States, despite their equivalent bars in this chart.

Figure 16. International Prescription Drug Prices as a Percentage of U.S. Prices, 1999.

Of course, price is only one part of the equation of a nation's spending on prescription drugs. Danzon and Furukawa found that the quantity of prescription drugs consumed in the United States is not markedly different from Canada, France and the United Kingdom, as shown in figure 17. However, the figure also demonstrates how much more the United States consumes of new drugs (two years old or newer). Still, even though the United States has the highest drug spending in the world, at $752 per person (figure 18), it is below the OECD average in terms of the percentage of health care spending devoted to pharmaceuticals (figure 19). The below-average results for prescription drugs suggest that U.S. spending on prescription drugs is not as high compared to the rest of the industrialized world as is its spending on other types of health care, as discussed in the following section.

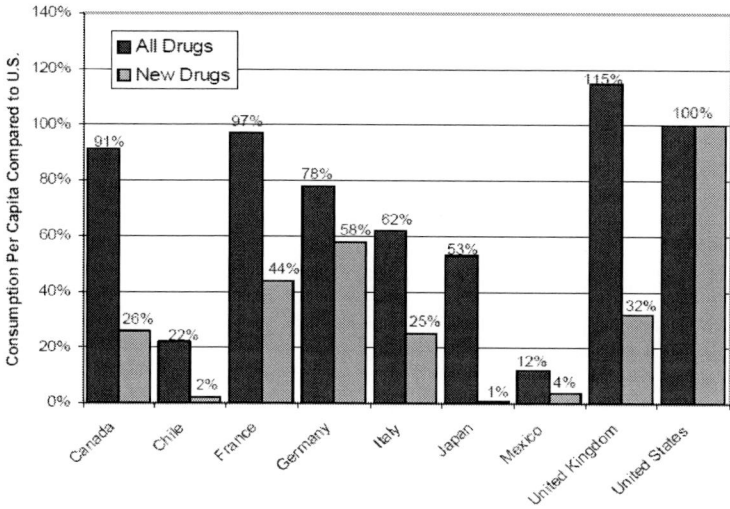

Source: Patricia M. Danzon and Michael F. Furukawa, "Prices and Availability of Pharmaceuticals: Evidence from Nine Countries," *Health Affairs,* Web exclusive, Oct. 29, 2003, pp. W3-521-W3-536, available at [http://content.healthaffairs.org/cgi/reprint/hlthaff.w3.521v1.pdf], Exhibit 7.

Notes: "New drugs" are those two years old or newer. From the 350 leading molecules (active ingredients) based on 1999 U.S. sales volume, Danzon and Furukawa chose 249 that were approved in at least four of the study countries or had been approved in the United States since 1992. All products with that active ingredient, including brand-name, generic, and over-the-counter products (if available), and all presentations (capsules, tablets) and strengths in each country were included. Note that consumption of new drugs and all drugs are not the same in the United States, despite their equivalent bars in this chart.

Figure 17. International Pharmaceutical Consumption as a Percentage of U.S. Consumption, for 249 Leading U.S. Molecules, 1999.

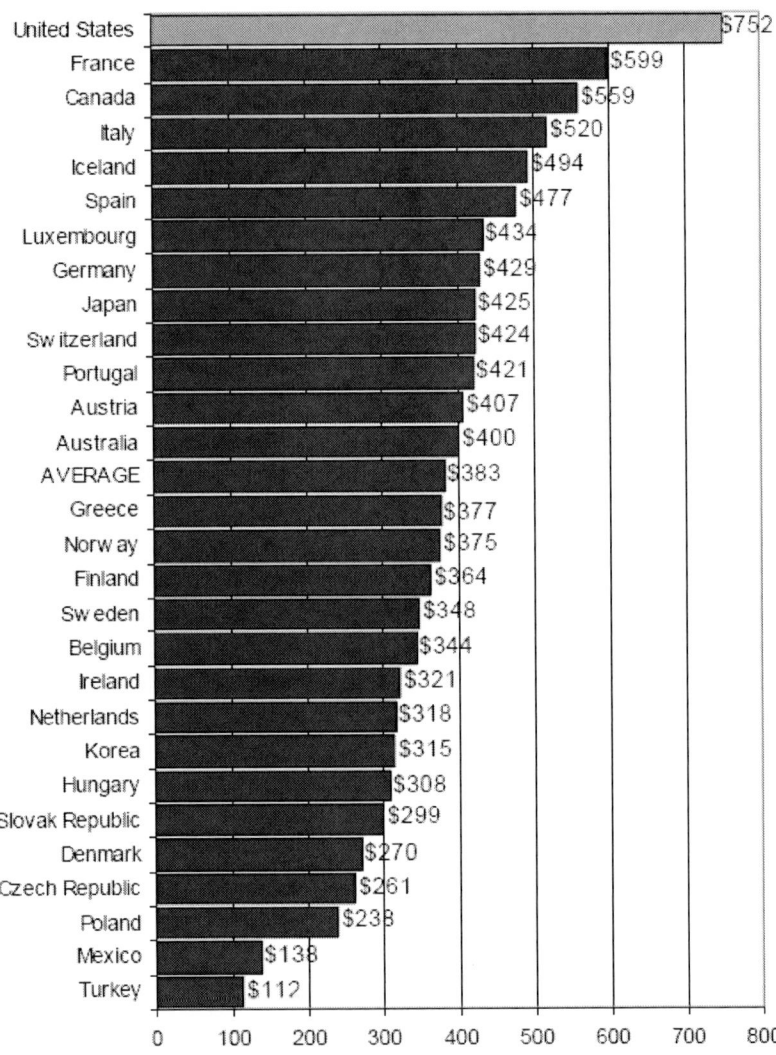

Notes: Amounts are adjusted using U.S. dollar purchasing power parities, and are based on estimates and/or earlier years for 16 countries: for Canada, Denmark, France, Iceland, Luxembourg, Portugal, Spain, Sweden, and Switzerland, amounts are 2004 estimates; for Belgium (estimate), Japan (estimate), and the Slovak Republic, the numbers are from 2003; for the Czech Republic, Hungary, and the Netherlands, amounts are from 2002; and for Turkey, amounts are from 2000. Recent data are available only for 28 of the 30 OECD countries.

Figure 18. Pharmaceutical Spending per Capita, 2004.

Price of Pharmaceuticals 47

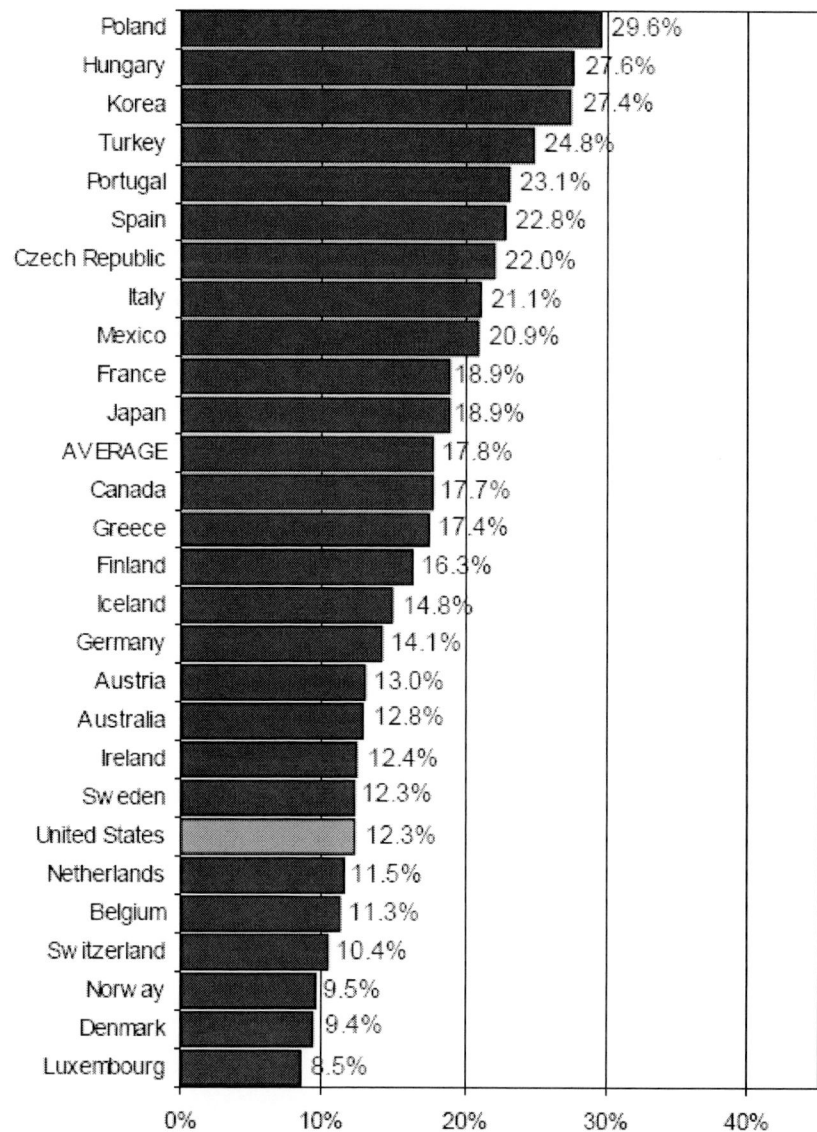

Notes: Amounts are based on spending in previous years for seven countries: for Belgium, Japan, and the Slovak Republic, the numbers are from 2003; for the Czech Republic, Hungary, and the Netherlands, the numbers are from 2002; and for Turkey, the numbers are from 2000. Recent data are available only for 27 of the 30 OECD countries.

Source: OECD Health Data 2006 (October 2006).

Figure 19. Pharmaceutical Spending as a Percentage of Total Health Spending, 2004.

Chapter 13

HEALTH CARE SPENDING BY TYPE OF SERVICE

Table 4 breaks down U.S. health care spending into component parts. For each of these components, the table shows the OECD median for the countries reporting the information and the U.S. rank for each category. In terms of the dollar amounts, U.S. spending was above the OECD median in every category in table 4 and the top spender on outpatient care, pharmaceuticals, and public health and prevention.

The largest dollar difference between the U.S. and the OECD median was in outpatient care; U.S. spending was $2,668 per person — three-and-a-half times the OECD median of $727. The U.S. level is almost double that of the second-highest spender in this category, Sweden ($1,381). However, the high level of U.S. outpatient spending may be driven partly by methodological issues.

In the United States, it is common for physicians to provide inpatient hospital care while not being employees of the hospital. For categorizing U.S. spending, these physician services are considered outpatient services, even though they are provided in an inpatient setting. The result is that the United States appears to have a higher proportion of outpatient spending and a lower proportion of inpatient spending than it otherwise would. Combined, however, outpatient *and* inpatient services account for 71% of spending in the United States, compared with 69% of spending in the median OECD country — quite similar percentages. Even so, total U.S. health spending per capita is still twice as high as the OECD average. If independently billing physician costs in the United States could be recategorized as inpatient spending, it is quite plausible that the United States would rank first in both outpatient and inpatient spending in table 4, with proportions of spending in-line with the other countries. This highlights yet again the care that must be taken when comparing international health expenditure data.[26]

Table 4. U.S. Health Care Expenditures per Capita, by Major Categories, Compared with Reporting OECD Countries, 2004

Expenditure	U.S.	OECD Median	U.S. Rank
Outpatient care	$2,668	$727	1 of 19
Inpatient care	$1,636	$1,061	4 of 19
Home health care	$147	$53	5 of 14
Ancillary services	NA	$133	NA of 13
Pharmaceuticals (non-durable medical goods)	$752	$407	1 of 21
Therapeutic appliances (durable medical goods)	$78	$76	9 of 18
Total personal health care	$5,280	$2,676	1 of 21
Prevention and public health	$224	$55	1 of 20
Health administration and insurance	$465	$66	2 of 21
Total collective health care	$689	$132	1 of 19
Total investment on medical facilities	$132	$101	7 of 26
TOTAL HEALTH CARE EXPENDITURES	$6,102	$2,596	1 of 27

Source: OECD Health Data 2006 (October 2006), with Congressional Research Service (CRS) calculations.

Notes: U.S. outpatient and inpatient amounts are not exactly comparable with the other OECD countries, because in the United States, costs generated by hospital physicians who independently bill are counted as outpatient care instead of inpatient care. Dollars are adjusted using U.S. dollar purchasing power parities. Medians are calculated based on the countries reporting the applicable information; "U.S. Rank" indicates the number of reporting countries. "N/A" means not available. "Therapeutic appliances" includes items like eyeglasses, hearing aids, and wheelchairs. "Ancillary services" include laboratory tests, diagnostic imaging, and patient transport. The United States does not report expenditures on ancillary services. Some countries report estimates instead of actual expenditures. A breakdown by category was not available for 11 countries (Belgium, the Czech Republic, Greece, Hungary, Ireland, Japan, the Netherlands, New Zealand, the Slovak Republic, Turkey, and the United Kingdom). Their median total per capita spending was $2,162, compared with $3,043 in the other 19 countries.

Health Care Spending by Type of Service 51

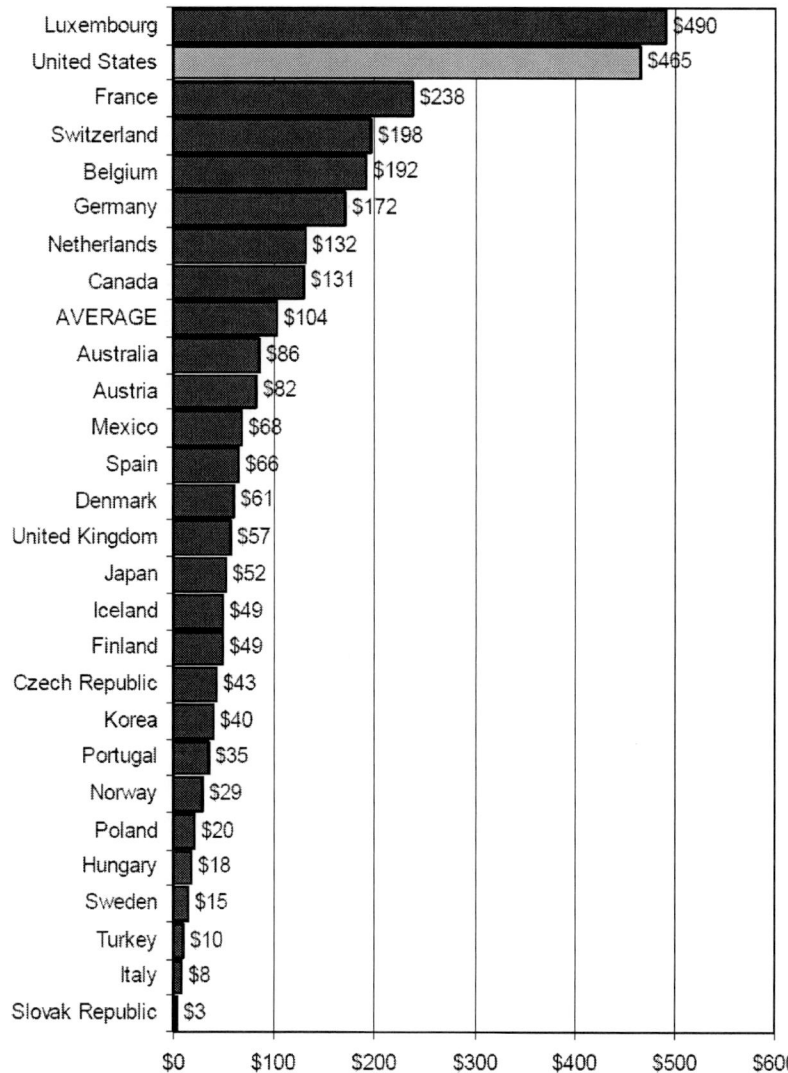

Source: OECD Health Data 2006 (October 2006).
Notes: Amounts are adjusted using U.S. dollar purchasing power parities, and are from a previous year for six countries: for Belgium, Japan, and the Slovak Republic, amounts are from 2003; for Hungary, the amount is from 2002; for Turkey, the amount is from 2000; and for the United Kingdom, the amount is from 1999. Recent data are available only for 27 of the 30 OECD countries.

Figure 20. Health Administration and Insurance Costs, 2004.

Spending on health administration and insurance in the United States ($465) was seven times that of the OECD median ($66), based on the 21 countries reporting the information in 2004. As a percentage of total health care spending, the United States (7.6%) was far above the OECD median (2.5%). The United States was outspent by only one country — Luxembourg ($490), which has two main types of private health insurance policies available to its 452,000 citizens: statutorily required, employer-sponsored private health insurance and voluntary supplemental health insurance policies (which cover 75% of the population yet pay out benefits worth only 2.2% of those paid out by the statutory plans).[27]

Spending on health insurance and administration can be broken into three parts. The largest part, at least in the United States, comprises the difference between earned premiums and incurred benefits of private health insurers. This difference accounts for insurers' administrative costs, net additions to reserves, rate credits and dividends, premium taxes, and profits or losses. The next largest part comprises the administrative expenses of government programs. The smallest part comprises the expenses associated with health activities of philanthropies. The complexity of the U.S. system may cause greater administrative costs within the other categories, but this is not quantified in the OECD data.

Chapter 14

WHAT SPURS HEALTH CARE PRICES AND UTILIZATION?

The preceding discussion described U.S. health care spending relative to most of the leading industrialized democracies. The discussion presented what information is available on the traditional components of spending: quantity (specifically, health care utilization in the form of volume and intensity) and price. However, price and quantity themselves are driven by even more fundamental factors, many of which have been alluded to already — for example, the population's health and income. Rather than dealing with a few of these factors piecemeal, this section uses what data are available to look more comprehensively at the factors that affect health care spending.

With a couple of exceptions that will be discussed, health care is similar in many respects to other goods and services that people purchase. For example, as prices drop, people tend to consume more. Using the classic supply-demand construct, health care has its suppliers (doctors, hospitals, pharmaceutical companies, etc.) and those who have a demand, or desire, to use health care (patients, consumers, etc.). This section describes many of the factors that can change the supply and the demand of health care, along with a discussion of their impact on price and utilization. Where possible, this section compares the impact of these factors in the United States with other OECD countries.

Chapter 15

FACTORS THAT AFFECT DEMAND

HEALTH

A population's health can affect the amount of health care they use. Determinants of health that are included in the OECD data are age (discussed in the next section), obesity, diet, and alcohol and tobacco consumption.

The incidence of certain diseases in a population can affect a nation's health care spending compared with others. However, the OECD data provide such information only for cancer (i.e., malignant neoplasms) and acquired immunodeficiency syndrome (AIDS). In both cases, the United States has the highest incidence in the OECD. In 2002, the incidence of cancer in the United States was 358 per 100,000 population, compared with the second-highest rate of 331 in New Zealand and the OECD average of 266. In 2002, the incidence of AIDS in the United States was 147 per 100,000 population, compared with the second-highest rate of 97 in Portugal and the OECD average of 19.

Using the available OECD data, if people in one country have greater rates of obesity than in another, one might expect them to have higher average health care spending. Although the OECD data provide estimates of the percentage of the population that is overweight and obese, only the United Kingdom uses a methodology similar to the United States. Both use actual measurements of people for their estimates. The other OECD countries use results from survey questions, which yields lower rates of obesity. In 2004, 34% of U.S. residents were estimated to be overweight (but not obese), compared with 39% of U.K. residents. However, the United States had a much greater percentage of its population that was considered obese (32%) than the United Kingdom (23%).

In lieu of comparable obesity data, information on populations' food consumption may also indicate their health and tendencies that lead to chronic, costly diseases such as diabetes and heart disease. The United States ranked first in both daily calorie consumption and annual sugar consumption per person in 2003 among OECD countries. U.S. sugar consumption was notably higher than all the other countries, at 156 pounds per person per year, compared with the OECD average of 99 pounds of sugar consumed per year.[28]

The United States had the 11th lowest rate of alcohol consumption. Among individuals aged 15 and older, average annual consumption of pure alcohol was 2.2 gallons in the United States, compared with the OECD average of 2.5 gallons and the top-ranked average in Luxembourg of 4.1 gallons.[29] The United States had the third-lowest percentage (17%) of daily smokers in 2004, after Canada (15%) and Sweden (16.2%). Greece had the highest percentage of daily smokers (39%).

The effects of obesity on health and health care spending have been found to be more serious than smoking or problem drinking — the effects of obesity are similar to 20 years' aging.[30] According to one estimate, 27% of the increase in per capita U.S. health care spending between 1987 and 2001 was attributable to obesity.[31] Another group of researchers estimated that 9.1% of total U.S. medical spending was attributable to obesity in 1998, with Medicare and Medicaid paying for half of these costs.[32] The OECD data do not provide estimates of how this might compare with other countries.

Chapter 16

AGE STRUCTURE OF THE POPULATION

Because the incidence of many of the most costly diseases tends to increase with age, the age structure of a population may also affect its per capita health care spending as compared with other nations. In the OECD countries, the percentage of the population aged 65 and older ranges from 6% in Turkey to 19% in Japan, Germany, and Italy. In the United States, 12% of the population was 65 and older in 2004, below the OECD average of 14%. In the United States, 26% of the population is 19 or younger, the seventh-highest in the OECD. Considering the strong association between age and health care spending, an aging population (although of concern within the United States) cannot be used as an explanation for this country's high health care spending relative to the rest of the world.

Chapter 17

INCOME

Changes in people's income shifts their demand for health care. As income increases, people tend to consume greater quantities of goods, such as health care, and are willing to pay higher prices. If people's incomes rise and the supply of products is not increased, then the price of those products would be expected to rise. As discussed earlier and illustrated in figure 2, a simple bivariate comparison suggests that varying GDP levels may account for 90% of the variation in per capita health care spending across the 30 OECD countries. Thus, one might expect the United States to have a high level of per capita health care spending compared with countries with a lower per capita GDP (although U.S. health care spending is still 60% higher than its GDP would predict).[33]

Chapter 18

INSURANCE

The presence of insurance also affects demand for health care. Because health insurance reduces people's out-of-pocket costs of care, people with health insurance will generally use more health care than people who lack insurance. The RAND Health Insurance Experiment, which took place in the 1970s and 1980s, found that those with a health insurance plan that covered *all* costs would seek nearly twice as much care as those with a health insurance plan that covered only 5% of the costs, with total spending directly related to the level of cost-sharing individuals faced.[34] The phenomenon of people seeking more (or any) health care because they face lower out-of-pocket costs from insurance is referred to in health economics as "moral hazard."[35] If the vast majority of Americans had health insurance that substantially lowered their out-of-pocket costs for health care, compared with people in other OECD countries, then the resulting increased utilization might arguably be attributed to moral hazard. However, this is not the picture that emerges.

First, the United States has the lowest percentage of its population enrolled in health insurance among those countries reporting. "The U.S. health care system is unique in the OECD area. The United States does not have a national insurance program and 14 percent of the population has no insurance coverage."[36] Twenty-two OECD countries provided 98% to 100% of their residents with public health insurance covering at least hospital and inpatient care in 2004.

The percentage of residents covered by public insurance in the other three countries reporting data for 2004 were as follows: 90% in Germany, 70% in the Netherlands, and 27% in the United States. Besides the United States, only the Netherlands' public health insurance coverage was below 90% among the 25 countries reporting. Including the Netherlands' private health insurance, "a very negligible portion of the population (less than 1%) remains uninsured."[37] Private health insurance increases U.S. coverage to 86% overall, still yielding the highest uninsured rate among the OECD countries reporting.[38] The OECD has noted that among its members only the United States, Mexico, and Turkey have not established "universal or near-universal coverage." "Mandatory/compulsory element (is) key to universality," according to the OECD.[39]

At first glance, with 45 million uninsured, moral hazard might appear not to contribute to high health spending in the United States. However, there is another factor affecting moral hazard besides simply coverage: Americans pay less out of pocket for care on average than the populations of most other OECD countries, which one might expect to lead to greater health care spending.

Specifically, as shown in figure 21, 13.2% of U.S. health care costs were paid by individuals out of their own pockets in 2004.[40] This is the fifth-lowest average rate of cost-sharing in the OECD, even including the effect of the uninsured. However, this is based on the *average* amount paid out of pocket, which obscures the variation in individuals' cost-sharing (e.g., some people who might be uninsured and face 100% cost-sharing, versus those with generous coverage who face little or no cost-sharing). More analyses are needed on the distribution of cost-sharing among countries' populations to more fully appreciate the impact of cost-sharing on overall health care spending.[41]

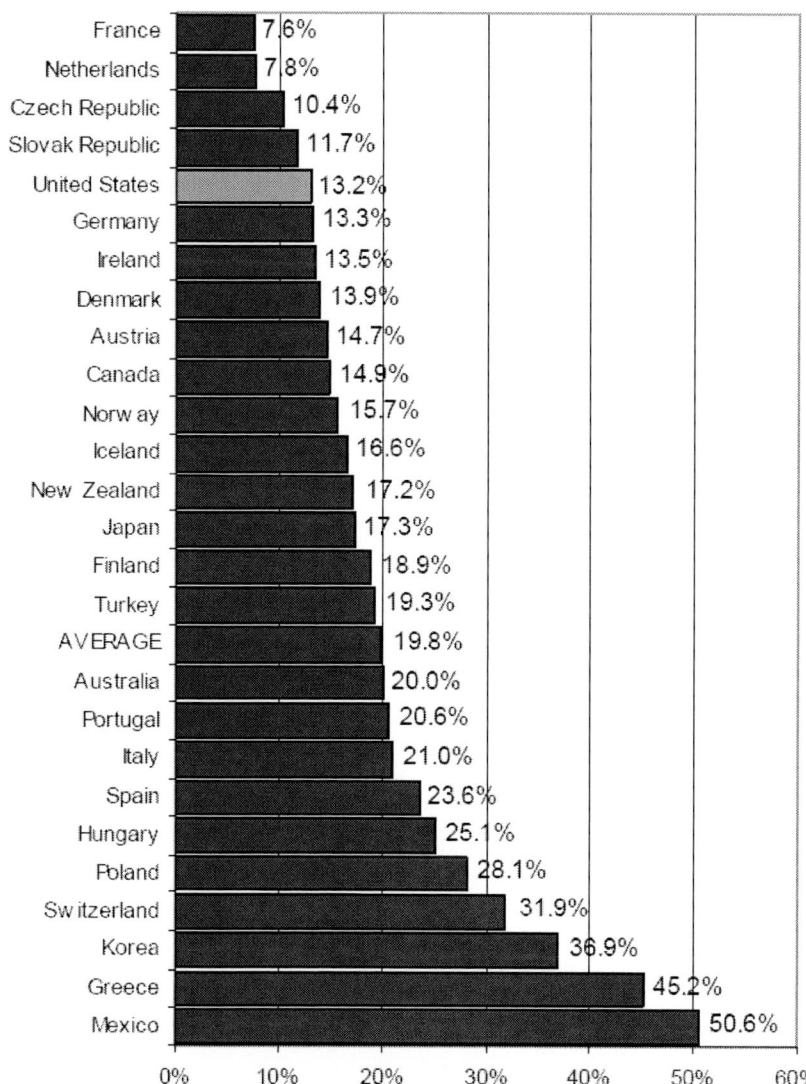

Source: OECD Health Data 2006 (October 2006).
Notes: Data are from a previous year for two countries: for the Slovak Republic, data are from 2003; for Japan, data are from 2002. Recent data are available only for 26 of the 30 OECD countries.

Figure 21. Percentage of Health Care Costs Paid Out-of-Pocket, 2004.

Chapter 19

TAX TREATMENT

Health insurance increases health care spending to the extent that it reduces the cost of services to individuals. The same is true for the tax treatment of health care costs and health insurance premiums. In the United States, wages set aside by employers to pay for health insurance are not subject to personal income tax. As a result, more money is available to pay for health insurance compared with the amount if it were paid out to workers, taxed, and then used to purchase coverage. When payments for health insurance premiums receive tax advantages, individuals tend to purchase richer health insurance benefits than they would in the absence of those tax benefits.[42]

In addition to tax preferences for employer-sponsored health insurance premiums, out-of-pocket health care costs are tax deductible once they exceed 7.5% of adjusted gross income (AGI) for those who itemize their tax returns. However, tax-advantaged accounts (for example, Health Savings Accounts) may enable some individuals to exempt *all* of their out-of-pocket health care costs from income tax —regardless of the amount of those expenses or whether or not individuals' tax returns are itemized. Premiums for non-group health insurance coverage (as opposed to employer-sponsored group coverage) are not tax deductible, except for the self-employed (and except to the extent that nongroup premiums contribute to exceeding 7.5% of AGI for individuals who itemize).[43]

In the United States, the forgone tax revenues resulting from federal tax policy are called tax expenditures. The cost of all health care-related tax expenditures was $141.5 billion in 2006, or $473 per person.[44] Some of these tax expenditures include tax exemption of employers' contributions for employee health insurance ($90.6 billion), deducting out-of-pocket medical expenses ($7.3 billion), and deducting health insurance premiums for the self-employed ($3.8 billion).[45] Unfortunately, a comparison of health-related tax expenditures across OECD countries is not available.

Chapter 20

TASTES

People's tastes can also affect demand for health care. Tastes for health care may be influenced by a variety of factors. A person's peers, or even culture, may encourage or discourage certain types of health care.[46] For example, one poll found that 34% of Americans thought that modern medicine could cure almost any illness, whereas only 27% of Canadians and 11% of Germans thought this.[47] It is possible that these attitudes may translate into greater reliance on advanced medical procedures by Americans.

Variation in attitudes toward health care also exist within the United States. In the Miami area, the average spending per Medicare beneficiary was $11,352 in 2003, compared with the national average of $6,611.[48] Some have suggested that this difference in spending is due to local expectations and patterns that are not attributable to local differences in population age, illness, or prices.[49]

Other external factors, such as advertising, may also affect tastes. Between 1996 and 2003, direct-to-consumer (DTC) advertising for prescription drugs more than quadrupled in the United States. A study by a pharmaceutical consulting firm found that 90% of the brands that were advertised DTC experienced a positive return on that investment. Seventy percent of the brands experienced returns in excess of $1.50 for every DTC dollar spent.[50] Other research suggests even higher returns.[51] Despite the fact that the United States is one of only two industrialized countries that allows direct-to-consumer advertising, whether U.S. health care spending overall is significantly affected by DTC advertising is debatable, let alone the extent to which its use and impact varies across the OECD.[52]

Chapter 21

WEAK BARGAINING POWER

Entities or individuals who purchase a relatively large amount of a good or service generally try to use that market power to obtain lower prices. As buying power becomes more diffuse, purchasers have reduced ability to obtain lower prices. Health care is no different. Insurers, representing thousands of people, are able to obtain lower prices for health care services; the uninsured, facing the market as individuals, often pay the highest prices. For example, one researcher found that uninsured individuals who were hospitalized for a heart attack were charged more than $30,000 on average, whereas the charge to insurance plans was less than $10,000.[53]

However, most Americans are covered by private health insurance and ostensibly receive care at lower prices than if they were uninsured. In addition, the publicly financed health insurance systems of Medicare and Medicaid do exert some buying power. However, some researchers note the potential impact of bargaining power:

> (T)he highly fragmented buy side of the U.S. health system is relatively weak by international standards. It is one factor, among others, that could explain the relatively high prices paid for health care and for health professionals in the United States. In comparison, the government-controlled health systems of Canada, Europe, and Japan allocate considerably more market power to the buy side. In each of the Canadian provinces, for example, the health insurance plans operated by the provincial governments constitute pure monopsonies: They purchase (pay for) all of the health services that are covered by the provincial health plan and used by the province's residents.[54]

Several years ago, U.S. insurers attempted to rein in costs with managed care. In the era that has followed, with the easing of managed care restrictions, plans have sought to rein in costs by other means. Since the late 1990s, "(p)lans' strategies centered on consolidation and geographic expansion, aggressive pricing to expand market share, and development of less restrictive managed care products."[55] Through acquisitions, there are now "megaplans" such as United Healthcare, which covers 65 million enrollees.[56] As of 2002-2003, the top three insurers in each state covered more than two-thirds of commercial insurance enrollees. In only three state markets did the top three insurers cover less than half of commercial insurance enrollees. However, the price effects of these consolidations have apparently been more than counterbalanced by consolidations on the supply side, as discussed in another section below.[57]

Having multiple health insurance plans creates increased administrative costs. As noted in table 4 and figure 21, the United States is the second-highest spender on health and insurance administration costs (at $465 per person), behind Luxembourg. However, this amount fails to capture spending by health care providers for their billing and insurance-related administration. These costs are discussed in the following section on the supply of health care.

Chapter 22

FACTORS THAT AFFECT SUPPLY

In addition to factors that can affect people's demand for health care, other factors can affect the quantity and type of health care services offered to patients. These supply factors can affect both price and utilization.

Chapter 23

SUPPLIER-INDUCED DEMAND

Supplier-induced demand is defined as the change in demand for health care "associated with the discretionary influence of providers, especially physicians, over their patients."[58] Some research suggests that when patients are faced with a choice of treatments for a condition, local medical practice patterns tend to determine which procedure is used more often.[59] In addition, researchers looking at the seemingly unexplained variation in Medicare spending across geographic areas came to the following conclusions:

> Regions and academic medical centers with greater overall spending rates ... is largely the result of the providers in these regions using more supply-sensitive care: more physician visits, hospitalizations, stays in ICUs, and diagnostic testing and imaging. The remarkable variation in the frequency of use of these services among regions demonstrates the role capacity plays. For example, rates of primary care visits vary by a factor of about three, visits to medical specialists by more than six, and hospitalizations for cancer, chronic lung disease and congestive heart failure by more than four.[60]

Over the years, these researchers have "consistently shown a positive association between the supply of staffed hospital beds and the rate of hospitalization for conditions that do not require surgery.... A similar relationship can be seen between the supply of physicians and visit rates, particularly for those specialties that spent most of their time treating chronic illness."[61] Research also indicates that, on average, the additional utilization and spending do not necessarily lead to better health outcomes.[62]

One study suggests that areas with new doctor-owned specialty cardiac hospitals see 200% faster growth in the number of heart procedures compared with areas with new cardiac programs at general hospitals. This research suggests that doctors' financial stakes in specialty hospitals cause them to refer more patients for surgery — especially relatively healthy patients.[63] There is also an extremely strong correlation between the number of acute hospital beds per capita and the number of acute care bed days per capita.[64] Even so, it is difficult to assess if the capacity is built to match demand, or the other way around. In terms of cross-country comparisons, OECD data do not demonstrate that supplier-induced demand and the payment incentives to health care providers drives U.S. health care spending above the rest of the world.

Chapter 24

SPECIALIST CARE EMPHASIS

In most Western industrialized countries, visits to generalists exceed the number of visits to specialists — but not in the United States, according to the OECD.[65] Conversely, some researchers concluded that areas with a greater supply of primary care physicians have lower rates of deaths, even after controlling for socioeconomic and demographic factors. One group of researchers remarked that "it is the relative roles of primary care physicians and specialists rather than their number that makes the difference in health outcomes."[66] Another study suggests that an increase in the number of general practitioners per population is associated with an increase in the quality of health care and reduced costs per patient.[67]

One study comparing elderly medical care in the United States and Canada found that Canadian seniors received 44% more evaluation and management services but 25% fewer surgical procedures than American seniors.[68]

A study comparing hospitals in Manhattan and Paris found that Manhattan hospitals saw 150% more hospital stays than Paris did for conditions that were considered to be preventable with appropriate primary care. There was less of a difference (20%) in the hospital rates for conditions that are not preventable through prior primary care. Because it also found that a higher proportion of Paris doctors practiced primary care (50%, compared with 30% of doctors in Manhattan), these researchers postulated that reduced use of primary care was causing increased use of hospitals for preventable conditions.[69]

Chapter 25

DEFENSIVE MEDICINE

Some have argued that U.S. physicians are more likely to practice defensive medicine — that is, ordering more tests or providing more care than they otherwise would in an attempt to avoid being sued for medical malpractice. In a recent survey of Pennsylvania physicians specializing in areas of medicine where litigation is frequent (such as surgeons, radiologists, and obstetricians/gynecologists), 93% reported practicing defensive medicine.[70] Quantifying the specific effect of defensive medicine on health spending is more difficult to measure. The most widely cited study on this issue indicated that states that adopted malpractice tort reforms reduced spending on two heart procedures (acute myocardial infarction and ischemic heart disease) by 5% to 9%.[71] However, a subsequent analysis by the Congressional Budget Office (CBO) that used a broader set of ailments found no effect of malpractice tort reform on health spending. It concluded that "[o]n the basis of existing studies and its own research, CBO believes that savings from reducing defensive medicine would be very small."[72] A more recent CBO analysis found that studies on the relationship between tort reforms and health spending are "inconsistent" and "mixed." CBO concluded that tort reforms are sometimes associated with higher health spending, sometimes lower spending, and sometimes no effect on health spending.[73]

Chapter 26

STRUCTURE OF HEALTH SYSTEM

The structure of a country's health system and providers' bargaining power has a major effect on a country's level of health spending. In the United States, many hospitals (and hospital systems) have consolidated in the past several years, enabling them to obtain better price leverage in negotiations of reimbursement rates with insurance plans. Available research indicates that this consolidation has enabled hospitals to obtain higher prices but has not led to demonstrable improvements in health care quality.[74] The numerous, evolving arrangements of health care providers make it difficult to define the current U.S. health care delivery system, let alone compare it with other countries, each with their own ongoing dynamics.

The OECD health system that differs most from the United States in terms of the structure is the United Kingdom. The United Kingdom has a government-run National Health Service (NHS), which not only pays directly for health expenses but employs the doctors and nurses that provide the care, as well as owns and operates most of the sites where that care is given. Various estimates put the U.K. National Health Service at the third or the fifth largest employer in the world.[75] As shown in table 2, in 2004 U.K. general practitioners were the second best-paid in the OECD, its nurses the third best-paid, and its specialists the sixth best-paid.

Health care makes up 8.1% of GDP in the United Kingdom, compared with 15.3% in the United States. As one OECD researcher noted, "Countries with single-payer systems or integrated public financing and delivery (national health services) found spending control easier."[76] For the NHS, this has been done using administered pricing, controls on the supply of health care, and specific budget limits. However, Simon Stevens, the British Prime Minister's health policy adviser from 1997 to 2004, said that the NHS had

> overly effective cost containment.... As a consequence, U.K. health care infrastructure was outdated, with old buildings and inadequate equipment. Britain had relatively few health professionals: two practicing physicians per 1,000 population

versus 2.8 in the United States and 3.3 in France and Germany. And it was undersupplying appropriate care, causing long waits for routine surgeries. These facts were reinforced by the growing tendency of the British media to substitute its long-standing stereotype of the NHS ("good") versus the U.S. health system ("bad"), with an equally polemical comparison of the NHS ("bad") with continental Europe ("good").

As a result, taxes were raised in 2003 in the U.K. with the explicit goal of raising the percentage of GDP attributable to health care.[77]

It is beyond the scope of this book to delve into a specific comparison of the U.K. and U.S. health care systems. However, the preceding discussion illustrates that the different characteristics of one system, which may initially appear advantageous, can also bring different challenges with which policy makers must grapple.

Earlier in this report, there was a discussion of insurers' administrative costs. Health care providers also face their own administrative costs, which include billing and insurance-related (BIR) functions. Although international comparisons of these costs are difficult, they have been included in comparisons between the United States and Canada, for example. One study found that "administration accounted for 31.0 percent of health care expenditures in the United States and 16.7 percent of health care expenditures in Canada." The researchers found that private health insurance administrative costs in the United States (13.2% of private health insurance expenditures) were not much higher than in Canada (11.7%). However, the greater Canadian reliance on public health insurance, with its lower administrative costs, was seen as being responsible for some of the overall differences. They also found that providers' administrative costs were lower in Canada.[78] A critic of this study has argued that the difference between these two countries' administrative costs should be calculated a different way, whereby overhead costs would be $572 higher in the United States than Canada, instead of $752 higher.[79]

Chapter 27

WHAT DOES THE UNITED STATES GET FOR ITS HEALTH CARE SPENDING?

This section presents study findings concerning certain outcomes in OECD health care systems. For the United States, many of the results are mixed. For example, in a study of five OECD countries (the United States, Canada, the United Kingdom., Australia, and New Zealand), no country emerged as clearly superior. The United States had the highest breast cancer survival rate but the lowest kidney transplant survival rate. In terms of preventable diseases, the United States had the highest prevalence of measles, but the lowest prevalence of Hepatitis B. In terms of process indicators, the United States had the highest rate of cervical cancer screenings.[80] Another survey found that higher proportions of Americans reported receiving recommended preventive services for diabetic and hypertensive patients compared with five other OECD countries. It also found that Americans were the least likely to have had the same doctor for five years or more, were most likely to complain that their doctor did not spend enough time with them, and were most likely to have left an appointment without getting important questions answered.[81]

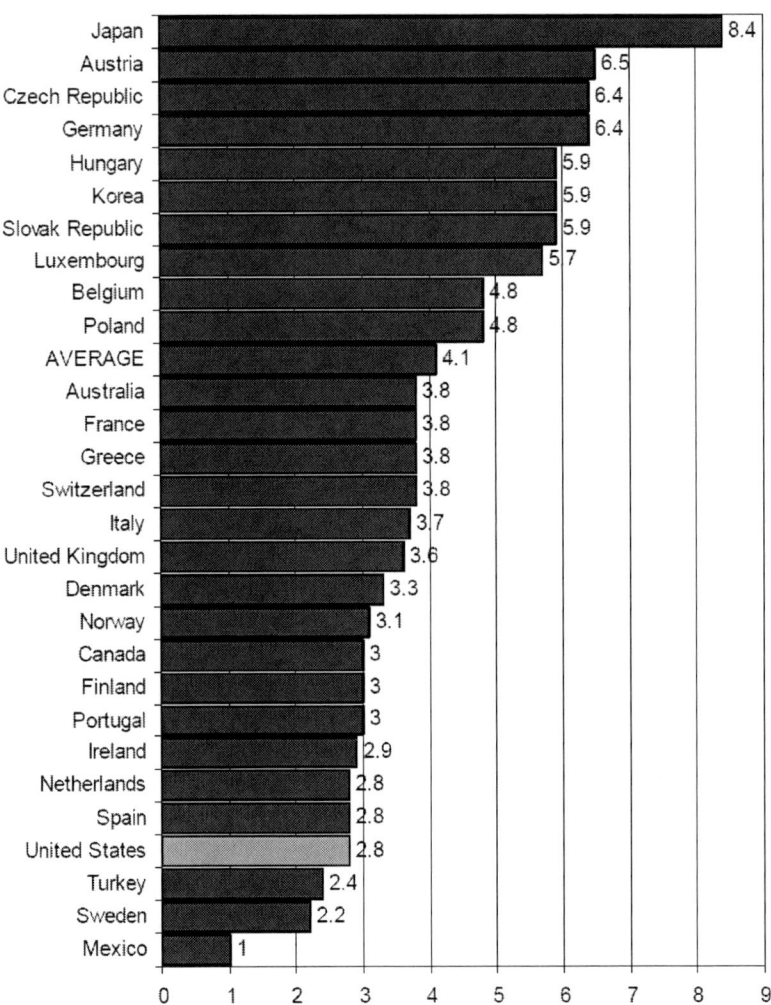

Source: OECD Health Data 2006 (October 2006).

Notes: Data for Canada, Denmark, Italy, Korea, the Netherlands, the Slovak Republic, and Spain are from 2003; data for Greece are from 2002. Recent data are available only for 28 of the 30 OECD countries.

Figure 22. Acute Care Hospital Beds per 1,000 Population, 2004.

A six-country comparison found that the United States was the best provider of preventive care but had the worst rating in terms of medical errors. This international survey of practitioners also found that the United States was fifth out of the six countries in terms of the "patient-centeredness" of care and the coordination of care between multiple providers. Patients in the United States were most likely to visit an emergency department for a condition that could have been treated by a regular doctor. However, once discharged, patients in the United States were less likely to be re-hospitalized because of complications than patients in four of the other countries. In the United States, records or test results were the least likely to reach a doctor's office in time for an appointment, and U.S. patients were more likely to be sent for duplicate tests compared with patients in four of the other countries.[82]

Chapter 28

WAIT TIMES

The United States is one of eight OECD countries in which waiting times for elective surgery are reported to be low. Meanwhile, wait times are considered a serious health policy issue in 12 OECD countries.[83] In these 12 countries, wait times of 1 to 1½ months are common for procedures such as invasive heart surgery, whereas wait times for procedures like hip or knee replacement cluster around five months. In a recent survey, a quarter to a third of respondents in Canada, the United Kingdom, and Australia reported waiting more than four months for a non-emergency procedure, compared with only 5% of Americans.[84]

Wait times are usually tied to capacity of the health care system, with low numbers of hospital beds and physicians typically associated with long wait times. Interestingly, the United States is the exception to this rule: here, low levels of beds and health care providers (figures 15 and 22) have not been accompanied by long wait times for elective surgery. International trends suggest that wait times are also associated with low total health spending; however, the exception to this rule is Japan, which spends only $2,249 on health per capita (compared with $6,102 in the United States) yet does not have a wait time problem. Wait times are more common in countries where physicians are paid by salary (such as in the United Kingdom) instead of on a fee-for-service basis (as in the United States).[85]

Although the United States does not have long wait times for non-emergency surgical procedures, this does not appear to be the case for primary care doctor visits. In a survey of five OECD countries in 2004, U.S. respondents were the second-least able to make a same-day doctor's appointment when sick and had the most difficulty getting care on nights and weekends. They were also the most likely to delay or forgo treatment because of cost.[86]

Chapter 29

SELF-REPORTED HEALTH STATUS

As shown in figure 23, 89% of Americans report their health as being "good," "very good," or "excellent" — the third highest levels in the OECD. Across OECD countries, there is a tendency for increased spending on health to accompany increased percentages of the population rating themselves as being in at least "good" health. However, countries that spend less than the United States on health care nevertheless enjoy similar high levels of reported health status. In particular, New Zealand, Ireland, and Canada spend a half to a third as much as the United States, yet the percentages of their populations who report a "good" or better health status is nearly identical to the United States.[87] These data are self-reported by individuals, so they may reflect differences in how people from different countries respond about their health status to such a survey, which may not reflect actual differences in individuals' health status.

Chapter 30

LIFE EXPECTANCY

The average life expectancy for a person in the United States is 77 ½ years — slightly below the OECD average, and 4½ years less than top-rated Japan (figure 24). Life expectancy is nearly 2½ years longer in Canada than in the United States. The United States is ranked 22nd out of 30 countries on life expectancy at birth, but once people reach the age of 65, U.S. life expectancy improves to a rank of 11th for men and 13th for women out of 30 countries reporting. Between 1960 and 2004, the United States gained 7.6 years of life expectancy — 2 years less than the OECD average of 9.7 years of additional life expectancy. Life expectancy tends to increase as countries spend more on health care per capita, except at very high levels of spending, as in the United States (figure 24).[88]

Chapter 31

MORTALITY RATES

The United States has a higher rate of deaths from natural causes than 17 OECD countries (table 5). The higher U.S. number of premature deaths (before the age of 70) from all causes except external causes (e.g., accidents) results in an average of 35.9 years of life lost per 1,000 people in the United States — a loss of roughly 7 additional years compared to the OECD average of 29 years of lost life per 1,000 people.

The top three causes of death in OECD countries are heart disease, cancer, and respiratory disease.[89] Death rates for heart disease in the United States are the 17th worst in the OECD, despite the fact that the United States performs substantially more invasive heart procedures than all other countries in the OECD (figure 9). However, since the OECD data do not provide the incidence of heart disease in the underlying population (which may be driven by more fundamental demographic characteristics), it is difficult to assess whether the death rates and frequency of certain procedures are appropriate or not.

As previously discussed, there are two diseases in the OECD for which incidence rates are provided: cancer and AIDS. In both cases, the incidence in the United States is higher than any other OECD country and well above the OECD average. Yet the United does *not* have the highest mortality rates for cancer or AIDS. For deaths resulting from cancer, the United States ranks 14th. For deaths resulting from AIDS, the United States ranks second (4.2 deaths per 100,000 population) behind Portugal (8.6).

In terms of respiratory diseases, the United States ranks 24th out of 30 countries, with twice as many people dying from respiratory diseases in the United States compared with the top-ranked countries, France, Switzerland, and Italy. Again, however, it is difficult to use this directly as a measure of a health care system's outcomes without knowing the incidence of respiratory diseases in the respective populations generally.

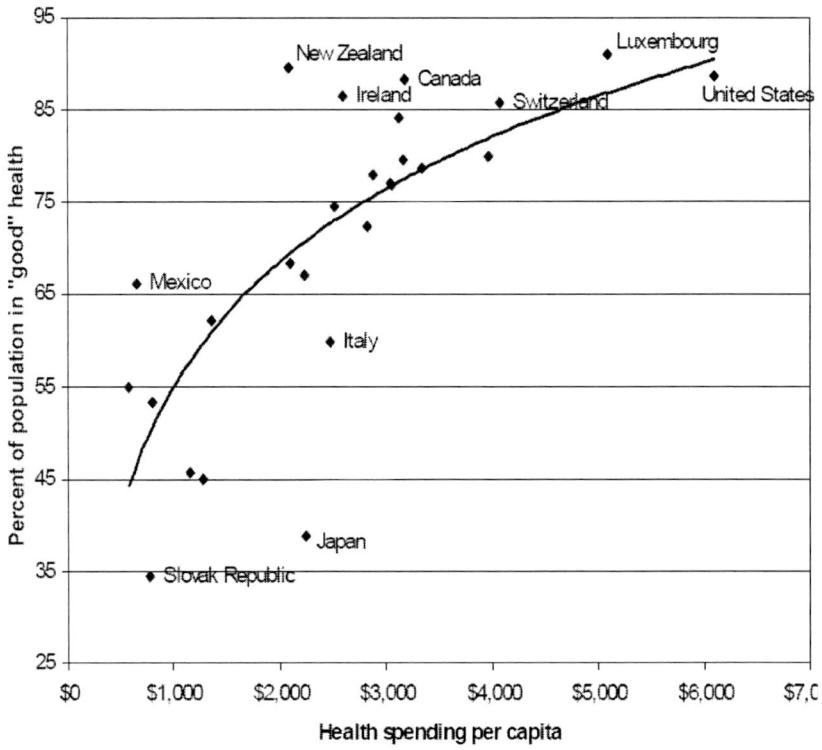

Source: OECD Health Data 2006 (October 2006).

Notes: "Good" health refers to people who reported their health status as being either "good," "very good," or "excellent." For Canada, Hungary, Ireland, Italy, New Zealand, the Slovak Republic, Spain, Turkey, and the United Kingdom, data are from 2003; for the Czech Republic, Mexico, Norway, and Switzerland, data are from 2002; for Korea, data are from 2001; and for Denmark, data are from 2000. Health care spending per capita is based on estimates or prior-year spending for 15 countries (Belgium, Canada, Czech Republic, Denmark, France, Greece, Iceland, Japan, Luxembourg, Netherlands, Portugal, Slovak Republic, Spain, Sweden and Switzerland). Dollars are adjusted for U.S. dollar purchasing power parity. R-squared of 0.55. Recent data are available only for 25 of the 30 OECD countries.

Figure 23. Health Spending per Capita and Self-Reported Health Status, 2004.

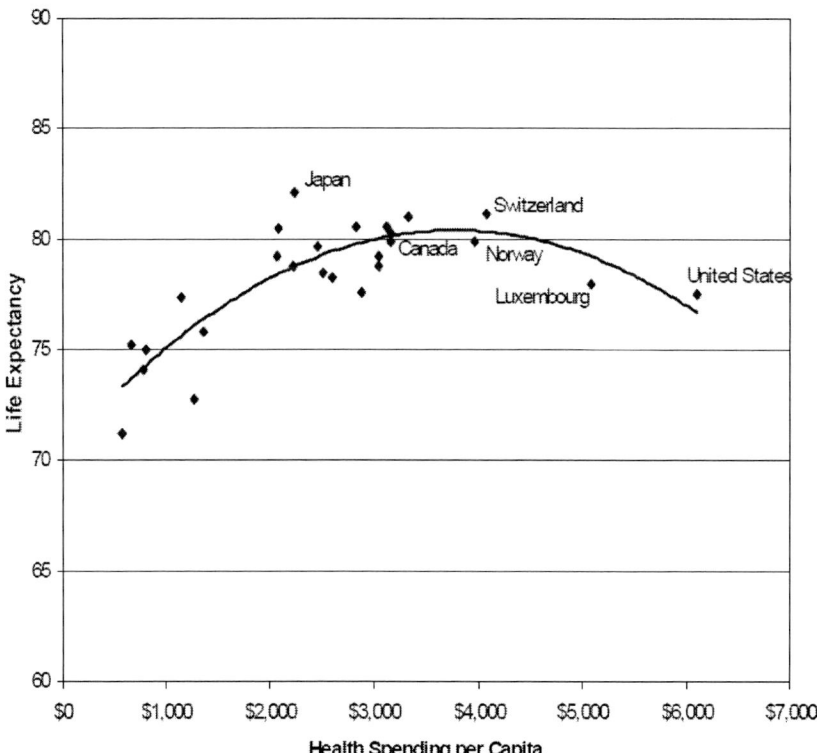

Source: OECD Health Data 2006 (October 2006).

Notes: Life expectancy data are from 2003 for seven countries: Ireland, Italy, Korea, Luxembourg, Portugal, United Kingdom, and the United States. Dollars are adjusted using U.S. dollar purchasing power parities. Health care spending per capita is based on estimates or prior-year spending for 15 countries (Belgium, Canada, Czech Republic, Denmark, France, Greece, Iceland, Japan, Luxembourg, Netherlands, Portugal, Slovak Republic, Spain, Sweden and Switzerland). Recent data are available only for 26 of the 30 OECD countries. The R-squared for this trendline is 0.73.

Figure 24. Health Spending per Capita and Life Expectancy, 2004.

Table 5. Life Expectancy and Mortality Rates, 2004

	Life expectancy at birth	Mortality rate (deaths per 1,000 people)	Potential years of life lost from natural causes, per 1,000 people
Japan	82.1	4.0	19.9
Switzerland	81.2	4.8	23.7
Iceland	81.0	4.8	16.8
Sweden	80.6	5.3	20.7
Australia	80.6	4.9	23.6
Spain	80.5	5.3	27.0
France	80.3	5.1	29.2
Norway	79.9	5.3	23.2
Canada	79.9	5.2	25.5
Italy	79.7	5.1	24.7
Austria	79.3	5.4	26.3
New Zealand	79.2	5.6	29.2
Netherlands	79.2	5.7	25.8
Greece	79.0	6.0	24.2
Finland	78.8	5.3	25.2
Belgium	78.8	N/A	N/A
Germany	78.6	5.6	27.1
United Kingdom	78.5	6.2	30.3
Ireland	78.3	6.5	29.5
Luxembourg	78.0	5.3	25.0
Denmark	77.6	6.7	30.7
United States	77.5	6.1	35.9
Portugal	77.4	6.4	33.8
Korea	77.4	6.4	30.7
Czech Republic	75.8	7.5	32.1
Mexico	75.2	N/A	N/A
Poland	75.0	7.8	43.1
Slovak Republic	74.1	8.6	45.3
Hungary	72.8	9.1	55.2
Turkey	71.2	N/A	N/A
AVERAGE	78.3	5.9	29.0

Source: OECD Health Data 2006 (October 2006).

Notes: Data sorted by life expectancy at birth. Mortality rate and potential years of life lost due to premature death do not include deaths from external causes. Potential years of life lost due to premature death is the sum of all deaths occurring at each age multiplied by the number of remaining years to live to age 70. "N/A" means not available. Data on life expectancy are from 2003 for seven countries: Ireland, Italy, Korea, Luxembourg, Portugal, United Kingdom, and the United States. Data on mortality rate are from previous years for all but six countries (Austria, the Czech Republic, Finland, Germany, Luxembourg, and the Netherlands): for Greece, Hungary, Iceland, Japan, Norway, Poland, Portugal, and Spain, the data are from 2003; for Australia, Canada, France, Ireland, Italy, Korea, the Slovak Republic, Sweden, Switzerland, the United Kingdom, and the United States, the data are from

2002; for Denmark, the data is from 2001; and for New Zealand, the data is from 2000. Data on potential years of lost life are from previous years for all but six countries (Austria, the Czech Republic, Finland, Germany, Luxembourg, and the Netherlands): for Greece, Hungary, Iceland, Japan, Norway, Poland, and Portugal, data are from 2003; for Australia, Canada, France, Ireland, Italy, Korea, the Slovak Republic, Spain, Sweden, Switzerland, the United Kingdom, and the United States, the data are from 2002; for Denmark, the data is from 2001; and for New Zealand, the data is from 2000.

Chapter 32

MEDICAL ERRORS

The United States has the third-highest rate of deaths from medical errors, among 26 countries reporting (figure 25). This poor ranking could be due to differences in reporting methodologies across OECD countries, higher rates of surgical procedures performed by doctors in the United States, or actual differences in the quality of medical care relative to other countries. In a 2004 poll, Americans were slightly more likely to report being given a wrong medication or dose (13%, compared with 9%-10% in the four other English-speaking OECD countries in the survey).[90]

Chapter 33

INFANT MORTALITY RATES

The United States has the third-highest infant mortality rate in the OECD, after Turkey and Mexico, as shown in figure 26. However, this statistic is likely somewhat overstated because of differences in methodology. The United States is one of eight countries that counts very premature babies with low chances of survival as "live births," which has the effect of increasing infant mortality rates over what they otherwise would be. Nevertheless, among the eight countries that report live births using the same methodology, the United States has the highest rate of infant mortality. Even with more consistent methodology, the U.S. ranking — which has been slipping over time — would probably not significantly improve.[91]

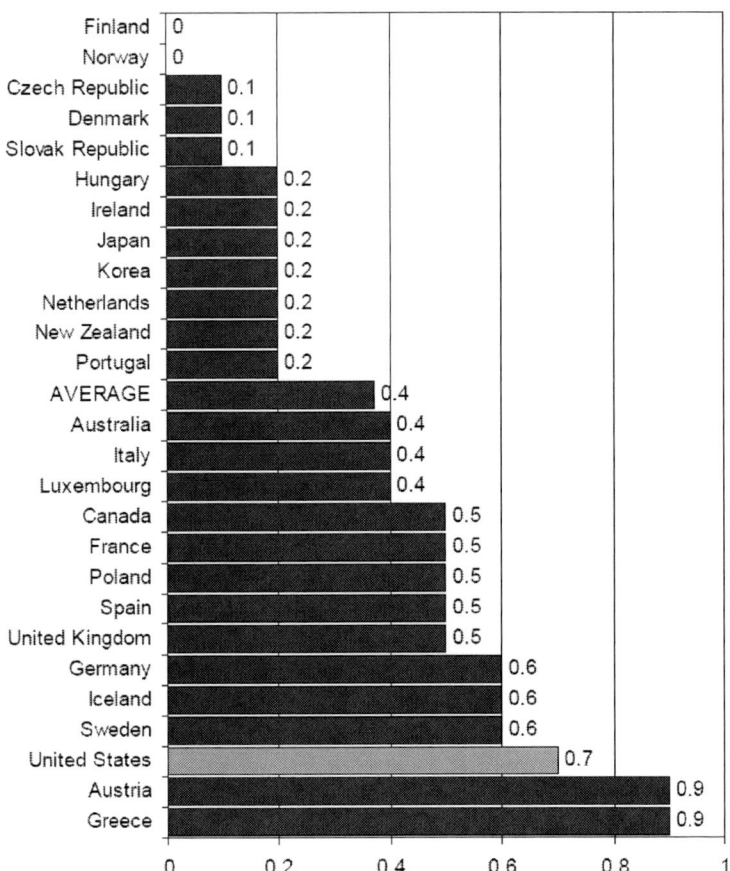

Source: OECD Health Data 2006 (October 2006).

Notes: Excludes surgical and medical procedures that are performed correctly but cause abnormal reactions in patients. Data for Greece, Hungary, Iceland, Japan, Norway, Poland, Portugal, and Spain are from 2003; for Australia, Canada, France, Ireland, Italy, Korea, the Slovak Republic, Sweden, the United Kingdom, and the United States, the data are from 2002; for Denmark, the data are from 2001; for New Zealand, the data are from 2000. Recent data are available only for 26 of the 30 OECD countries. The reported differences could be due to differences in reporting methodologies across the OECD, higher rates of surgeries performed by doctors in some countries, or actual differences in care.

Figure 25. Deaths from Medical Errors per 100,000 Population, 2004.

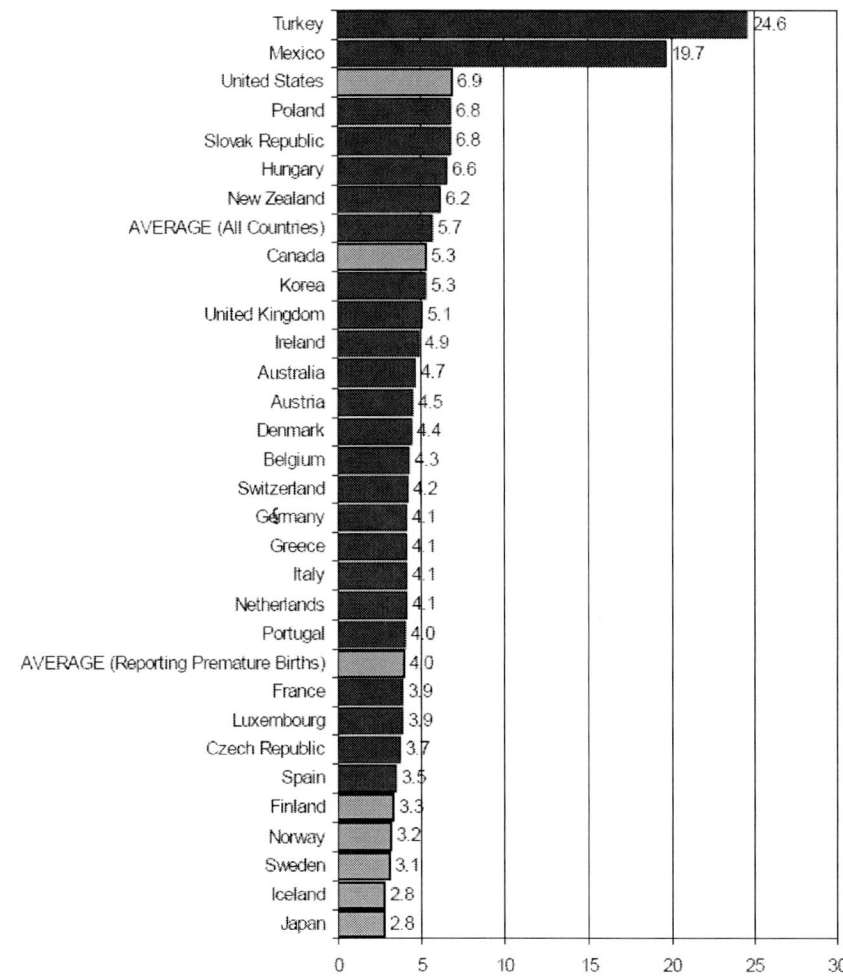

Source: OECD Health Data 2006 (October 2006).

Notes: Infant mortality rate is the number of deaths of children who are under one year of age, expressed per 1,000 live births. OECD countries differ in how they calculate the number of live births: countries represented by light shaded bars register very premature babies with low odds of survival as live births (Canada, Denmark, Finland, Iceland, Japan, Norway, Sweden, and the United States); countries represented by dark shaded bars do not count these as live births. Numbers are from a previous year for four countries: for Canada and the United States, data are from 2003; for Korea and New Zealand, data are from 2002.

Figure 26. Infant Mortality Rates per 1,000 Live Births, 2004.

Chapter 34

DOES THE UNITED STATES SPEND "TOO MUCH" ON HEALTH CARE?

Health economists are divided over whether the amount the United States spends on health care is "too much." Some economists have produced cost-benefit analyses finding that increased life expectancy and better health have been "worth the increased cost of care."[92] Researchers also determined that, with respect to the seven years of additional life expectancy gained between 1960 and 2000, an average of $19,900 was spent per year of life gained. They concluded that "the increases in medical spending since 1960 have provided reasonable value."[93] However, the amount spent per year of life gained varied depending on the decade and the age cohort. For example, the average cost of each year of life gained for individuals 65 and older was $145,000 between 1990 and 2000, which the authors indicated "fails to meet many cost-benefit criteria."[94]

Others have argued that just because benefits exceed costs does not mean U.S. health dollars are being spent as efficiently as they could be. Because the average OECD country experienced larger gains in life expectancy than the United States between 1960 and 2000 while spending less than the United States on health care, these countries would presumably have larger benefit-cost ratios using the above methodology. Some economists have pointed to studies finding that higher-cost, higher-intensity care is not associated with better health outcomes for Medicare patients.[95] Several have used the term "flat-of-the-curve medicine" to characterize much of the care provided in the United States, referring to the practice of providing extra medical care that provides little or no additional health benefit.[96] Others have argued that when the government is paying the bill (as in the Medicare program), providers should be required to practice more cost-effective medicine, based on an independent organization's assessments of the cost-effectiveness of clinical interventions.[97] Finally, another group of economists have argued that increases in health spending can actually be harmful to national health, because as spending rises, the cost of health insurance premiums also go up — making it harder for people to afford coverage and to get access to care.[98]

Rising health spending is occurring not only in the United States but also in the vast majority of OECD countries. U.S. growth in health spending was more than double inflation in 2004, at 6.9%, but this was not much higher than the OECD average rate of growth, at 6.2%. Over the longer term, health spending between 1970 and 2002 grew slightly faster in the United States (4.3% annually) than the average OECD country (3.8% annually, among 20 high-income OECD countries studied).

One study by an analyst from CBO broke down growth in health spending into three parts: growth resulting from a country's population aging; growth resulting from increases in economic growth; and "excess growth."[99] That analysis suggested that, from 1970 to 2002, the United States had below-average aging growth and economic growth, but nearly double the "excess growth" compared with the 20-country OECD average (figure 27). Over time, the rate of annual excess growth had remained essentially unchanged in the United States, according to that analysis, but had dropped substantially in other OECD counties. The author stated the following:

> "Those countries using public-integrated and public-contract financing models might have had more success in constraining spending than the United States has had. The United States, outside of Medicare, does not use a centralized authority to set health spending budgets or negotiate prices with providers, and this could contribute to a relative lack of spending constraint. Perhaps because of their relative success in constraining costs, the health care reforms currently under way in the OECD are no longer generally focused on cost constraint and are instead focused on quality of care, output and efficiency in the production of health care services, and responsiveness to patients' needs."[100]

Historically, growth in health spending in the United States has been accompanied by increases in the share of health spending that is publicly financed (from 25% in 1960 to 45% in 2005) and a lowering of the proportion of health spending that is paid out-of-pocket (from 47% in 1960 to 12.5% in 2005).[101] It may be reasonable to expect these trends to continue, if growth in health spending persists at its current pace.

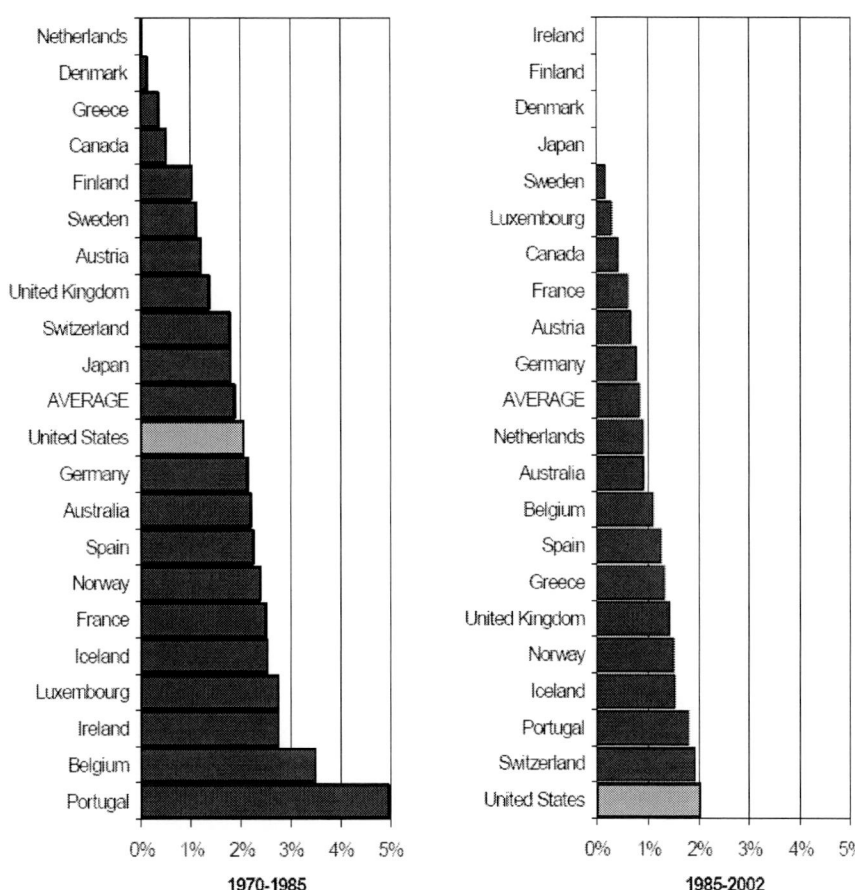

Source: Chapin White, "Health Care Spending Growth: How Different Is The United States From The Rest Of The OECD?" *Health Affairs*, 2007, vol. 26, no. 1, pp. 154-161, available at [http://healthaff.highwire.org/cgi/reprint/26/1/154], subscription required.

Notes: For the 1985-2002 period, three countries had negative rates of excess growth (not shown): Ireland (-0.6%), Finland (-0.4%), and Denmark (-0.1%).

Figure 27. Annual "Excess Growth" (Growth Not Attributable to Demographic or Economic Changes) in Health Spending per Capita, 1970-1985 and 1985-2002.

Chapter 35

CONCLUSION

SUMMARY OF FINDINGS

Total Spending

In 2004, the United States spent more than twice as much on health care as the average OECD country, at $6,102 per person (compared with the OECD average of $2,560). Health care spending comprised 15.3% of the U.S. GDP in 2004, compared with an average of 8.9% for the average OECD country (figure 1). Although a country's health expenditures are highly correlated with GDP (figure 2), U.S. health spending is nevertheless 60% greater than its GDP alone would predict.

Chapter 36

HEALTH CARE RESOURCES

The United States has fewer hospital admissions (figure 3) and doctor visits (figure 4) than the average OECD country. The United States has a below-average number of hospital beds (figure 22) and practicing physicians per population (figure 15), but its number of nurses per population is roughly the same as the OECD average. The United States has a higher than average number of staff per hospital bed (figure 10) and nurses per bed (figure 11). The length of hospital stays in the United States are the same as the OECD average (figure 5).

The United States spent a per capita average of $2,668 on outpatient care in 2004 — three-and-a-half times the OECD average. In most OECD countries, visits to general practitioners outnumber visits to specialists — but not in the United States. The United States has a greater supply of advanced technological equipment than other OECD countries, with nearly twice as many CT scanners per capita as the OECD average (figure 12) and three times as many MRI machines (figure 13). The United States also performs far more heart procedures per population than the average OECD country (figure 9), and an above-average amount of organ transplants per capita, but does not perform more of *all* types of surgical procedures.

Chapter 37

Pharmaceuticals

The United States spends more on prescription drugs per capita than any other OECD country (figure 18). The United States also *consumes* more prescription drugs than most OECD countries, according to a nine-country study (figure 17). That study found that the United States paid more for brand name drugs but less for generic drugs than other OECD countries (figure 16).

Chapter 38

HEALTH ADMINISTRATION AND INSURANCE

Spending on health administration and insurance cost $465 per person in the United States in 2004, which was seven times that of the OECD median (figure 20). Americans pay less out-of-pocket for health care (as a percentage of total health care spending) than residents of most OECD countries (figure 21).

Chapter 39

PRICES

Although OECD data does not compare prices of medical care, other studies have found that the United States pays higher prices for medical care than countries such as Canada and Germany. Part of the reason for this may be that U.S. general practitioners and nurses are the highest paid in the OECD, and U.S. specialists are the third-highest paid in the OECD (table 2). Health professionals in wealthier countries earn higher salaries than those in poorer countries (figure 14), but even accounting for this, U.S. health professionals are paid significantly more than the U.S. GDP would predict (for example, specialists are paid approximately $50,000 more than would be expected). However, U.S. health care professionals also enter the careers with substantially more educational debt than in other OECD countries. For example, in 2006, 62% of new U.S. medical school graduates had educational debt exceeding $100,000.[102]

Chapter 40

POPULATION RISK FACTORS

The United States had a lower than average proportion of the population that is elderly in 2004, and lower than average rates of smoking and drinking. The United States consumes more calories and sugar per capita than any other OECD country: the United States consumes 156 pounds of sugar per person per year, compared with 99 pounds in the average OECD country. In 2004, 34% of Americans were overweight and an additional 32% were obese. Obesity is associated with a 77% increase in consumption of medications and a 36% increase in inpatient and outpatient spending, according to one study.

Chapter 41

QUALITY

In terms of quality of health care, a five-country study found that each of the five countries studied (the United States, Canada, the United Kingdom, Australia, and New Zealand) had the best and worst health outcomes on at least one measure, but no country emerged as a clear quality leader. For example, the United States had the highest breast cancer survival rate but the lowest kidney transplant survival rate. A six-country study (the United States, Canada, the United Kingdom, Australia, New Zealand, and Germany) found that Americans were most likely to report receiving specific recommended preventive services for diabetic and hypertensive patients, but were most likely to complain that their doctor did not spend enough time with them and did not have a chance to answer all of their questions.

Chapter 42

WAIT TIMES

The United States is one of eight countries in which wait times for elective surgery are reported to be low. In a recent survey, a quarter to a third of respondents in Canada, the United Kingdom, and Australia reported waiting more than four months for a non-emergency procedure, compared with only 5% of Americans. In terms of doctor visits to primary care physicians, a five-country survey found that Americans had the greatest difficulty getting care on nights and weekends and were the most likely to forgo care because of cost.

Chapter 43

HEALTH OUTCOMES

The United States has the third-highest percentage of the population that reports their health status as being "good," "very good," or "excellent" (figure 23). However, the United States has below-average life expectancy (figure 24) and mortality rates (table 5). The United States has the third-highest rate of deaths from medical errors (figure 25) and the highest infant mortality rate among the eight countries that report this metric similarly (figure 26). However, such measures are often subjective or limited by differing measurement methodologies. They may also reflect fundamental population differences (in underlying health, for example) rather than differences in countries' health care systems. These are just some of the difficult research issues facing international comparisons like those used in this report.

REFERENCES

[1] The OECD Health Data 2006, from October 2006, provides much of the data for this report. Most of the data in this report are from 2004, the most recent year in which most countries provided data. For more information about the OECD, see CRS Report RS21128, *The Organization for Economic Cooperation and Development*, by James K. Jackson. Unless otherwise noted, the United States is included when calculating OECD averages.

[2] Uwe Reinhardt et al., "U.S. Health Care Spending in an International Context," *Health Affairs*, vol., 23, no. 3, May/June 2004, p. 24, available at [http://content.healthaffairs. org/cgi/reprint/23/3/10.pdf].

[3] The OECD defines per capita doctor visits as ambulatory contacts with physicians (both generalists and specialists) divided by the entire population. The number of contacts normally includes visits of patients at the physician's office, in primary care clinics and in outpatient departments of hospitals, and visits made to the patient's home.

[4] Acute care refers to curative care, typically provided in hospitals. The other type of hospital care measured in OECD data is long-term care, usually provided in nursing homes.

[5] In the OECD data, the United States ranked near or at the bottom in terms of its average length of hospital stays for most diagnostic categories. The notable exceptions were for perinatal conditions (e.g., conditions requiring care in a neo-natal intensive care unit (NICU)), in which the U.S. ranked 7th, and congenital abnormalities, in which the U.S. ranked 10th. Although the United States had the seventh-highest length of hospital stay for perinatal conditions, it had the fourth-*lowest* number of hospital discharges for these conditions. In other words, the United States had relatively fewer individuals hospitalized for perinatal conditions, but those who were hospitalized had relatively long stays.

[6] Naoki Ikegami et al., "Applying RUG-III in Japanese long-term care facilities," *The Gerontologist*, 1994, vol. 34, no. 5, pp. 628-639.

[7] The exception is lung transplants, for which the United States was ranked ninth among reporting OECD countries in 2003 in terms of the number of transplants performed per 100,000 people in the population.

[8] The conditions that the United States performed more frequently were coronary angioplasties (including stenting), coronary bypass grafts, cardiac catheterizations, implanting pacemakers, hysterectomies, and knee replacements. The conditions that the United States performed less frequently were appendectomies, prostatectomy, hip replacements, and mastectomies. The United States performed more organ transplants than the OECD median for all six types of transplants: bone marrow, heart, liver, lung, kidney, and functioning kidney. Medians are used in these cases because single outlier cases substantially skew the averages.

[9] Note that some countries calculate this measure based on number of full-time equivalent staff, while others use a head count. Data for the United States use full-time equivalent staff, but do not match the OECD definition.

[10] Naoki Ikegami and John Creighton Campbell, "Japan's Health Care System: Containing Costs and Attempting Reform," *Health Affairs*, May/June 2004, vol. 23, no. 3, pp. 26-36, available at [http://content.healthaffairs.org/cgi/reprint/23/3/26].

[11] James Lubitz, "Health, Technology, And Medical Care Spending," *Health Affairs*, Web exclusive, September 26, 2005, pp. W5-R81-W5-R85, available at [http://content. healthaffairs.org/cgi/reprint/hlthaff.w5.r81v1.pdf].

[12] John E. Wennberg et al., "Geography and the Debate Over Medicare Reform," *Health Affairs*, Web exclusive, February 13, 2002, pp. W96-W114, available at [http://content.healthaffairs.org/cgi/reprint/hlthaff.w2.96v1.pdf].

[13] Jonathan Skinner and John E. Wennberg, "Exceptionalism Or Extravagance? What's Different About Health Care In South Florida," *Health Affairs*, Web exclusive, August 13 2003, pp. W3-372-W3-375, available at [http://content. healthaffairs.org/cgi/reprint/hlthaff. w3.372v1.pdf].

[14] Gerard Anderson et al., "It's the Prices, Stupid: Why The United States Is So Different From Other Countries," *Health Affairs*, May/June 2003, vol. 22, no. 3, pp. 89-105, available at [http://content.healthaffairs.org/cgi/reprint/22/3/89.pdf].

[15] Elizabeth Docteur et al., *The US Health System: An Assessment and Prospective Directions for Reform*, OECD Economics Department Working Paper No. 350, available at [http://www.oecdwash.org/PDFILES/us_health_ecowp350.pdf].

[16] Association of American Medical Colleges, "2006 Medical School Graduation Questionnaire: All Schools Report, Final," p. 49, available at [http://www.aamc.org/data/gq/allschoolsreports/2006.pdf].

[17] John Antoniou et al., "In-Hospital Cost of Total Hip Arthroplasty in Canada and the United States," *Journal of Bone and Joint Surgery*, November 2004, vol. 86, no. 11, pp. 2435-2439.

[18] M.J. Eisenberg et al., "Outcomes and cost of coronary artery bypass graft surgery in the United States and Canada," *Archives of Internal Medicine*, 2005, vol. 165, no. 13, pp. 1506-1513.

[19] Anya C. Brox et al., "In-hospital cost of abdominal aortic aneurysm repair in Canada and the United States," *Archives of Internal Medicine*, November 10, 2003, vol. 163, no. 20, p. 2500.

[20] "Prescription Drugs: Companies Typically Charge More in the United States Than in Canada," General Accounting Office (GAO) Report HRD92-110, September 1992, available at [http://archive.gao.gov/d35t11/147823.pdf]; "Prescription Drugs: Companies Typically Charge More in the United States Than in the United Kingdom," General Accounting Office (GAO) Report HEHS-94-29, January 1994, available at [http://archive.gao.gov/t2pbat4/150655.pdf].

[21] For these reports, "price" was the amount paid by wholesalers to drug manufacturers.

[22] More generally, "international drug price comparisons are extremely sensitive to choices made about certain key methodological issues, such as sample selection, unit of measurement for price and volume, the relative weight given to consumption patterns in the countries being compared, and the use of exchange rates or purchasing power parities for currency conversion." Patricia M. Danzon and Jeong D. Kim, "International Price Comparisons for Pharmaceuticals: Measurement and Policy Issues," *Pharmacoeconomics*, 1998, 14 Suppl. 1, pp. 115-128, available at [http://hc.wharton. upenn.edu/danzon/PDF% 20Files/Intl%20Price%20Comparisons%20for%20Pharma_Mar98%20Pharmac oEcon.pdf].

[23] Patricia M. Danzon and Michael F. Furukawa, "Prices and Availability of Pharmaceuticals: Evidence from Nine Countries," *Health Affairs* Web exclusive, October 29, 2003, pp. W3-521-36, available at [http://content. healthaffairs.org/cgi/reprint/ hlthaff.w3.521v1.pdf]. The numbers represent the wholesale list prices (that is, the amount charged by manufacturers to wholesalers). The numbers also incorporate the authors' estimates of "off-invoice discounts," which reduced U.S. prices by approximately 8%. The comparisons are based on currency exchange rates rather than PPPs because currency exchange rates will be the basis of manufacturers' decisions when projecting their sales revenue.

[24] Research by the government of Australia suggests that the price of generics in the United States is not as low compared with other countries as the Danzon and Furukawa research indicates. However, the Australia report was intended for comparing other countries' drug prices with Australia alone, not to each other. Methodological issues makes cross-country comparisons for the Australia

report problematic. "As the bilateral comparisons are based on Australian consumption patterns and different bundles of pharmaceuticals for each country comparison with Australia, conclusions about relative price levels across countries cannot be drawn" (Productivity Commission 2001, *International Pharmaceutical Price Differences*, Research Report, AusInfo, Canberra, available at [http://www.pc.gov.au/study/ pbsprices/finalreport/pbsprices.pdf]).

[25] Malcolm Gladwell, "High Prices," *The New Yorker*, October 25, 2004, vol. 80, no. 32, p. 86, available at [http://www.gladwell.com/ 2004/2004_ 10_25_a_ drugs.html].

[26] The categories of U.S. health care expenditures are available at [http://www.cms.hhs.gov/ NationalHealthExpendData/downloads/quickref.pdf]. For additional information, see "Note on General Comparability of Health Expenditure and Finance Data in OECD Health Data 2005," [http://www.irdes.fr/ecosante/ OCDE/411.html], which also provides a link to country-specific definitions.

[27] Elizabeth Kerr,"Health Care Systems in Transition: Luxembourg," European Observatory on Health Care Systems, 1999, available at [http://www.euro. who.int/document/ e67498.pdf].

[28] OECD data is reported in kilograms, and has been converted to pounds in this report. The United States ranked 7th in annual per capita consumption of fat, 6th in consumption of protein, and 12th in consumption of fruits and vegetables.

[29] OECD data is reported in liters and has been converted into gallons in this report.

[30] Roland Sturm, "The Effects of Obesity, Smoking, and Drinking on Medical Problems and Costs," *Health Affairs*, March/April 2002, vol. 21, no. 2, pp. 245-53, available at [http://content.healthaffairs.org/cgi/reprint/21/2/245.pdf].

[31] Kenneth E. Thorpe et al., "The Impact of Obesity on Rising Medical Spending," *Health Affairs,* Web exclusive, October 20, 2004, pp. W4-480-486, available at [http://content.healthaffairs.org/cgi/reprint/hlthaff.w4.480v1.pdf].

[32] Eric Finkelstein, Iam Fiebelkorn, and Guijing Wang, "National Medical Spending Attributable To Overweight And Obesity: How Much, And Who's Paying?" *Health Affairs*, Web exclusive, May 14, 2003, pp. W3-219-W3-226, available at [http://content.healthaffairs.org/cgi/reprint/hlthaff.w3.219v1.pdf].

[33] Health care is what economists call a "luxury good," because richer people (and nations) buy it in greater proportions (see, for example, W.J. Moore et al., "Measuring the Relationship between Income and National Health Expenditures,"*Health Care Financing Review* 14, no. 1, 1992, pp. 133–139). For example, as GDP per capita rises, the percentage of GDP devoted to health care also rises. (If health care were a "normal good," the percentage of a nation's GDP devoted to health would not change when GDP per capita

increased.) Even so, the United States' GDP per capita predicts that health care would comprise 10% of GDP rather than 15%.

[34] Joseph P. Newhouse et al., *Free for All? Lessons from the RAND Health Insurance Experiment* (Cambridge, Massachusetts: Harvard University Press, 1993), Table 4.17. "For most people enrolled in the RAND experiment, who were typical of Americans covered by employment-based insurance, the variation in use across the plans appeared to have minimal to no effects on health status. By contrast, for those who were both poor and sick — people who might be found among those covered by Medicaid or lacking insurance — the reduction in use was harmful, on average. In particular, hypertension was less well controlled among that group, sufficiently so that the annual likelihood of death in that group rose approximately 10 percent. This adverse effect occurred in spite of the reduced cost sharing for low-income families, a feature generally not found in today's plans." (Joseph P. Newhouse, "Consumer-Directed Health Plans And The RAND Health Insurance Experiment," *Health Affairs*, vol. 23, no. 6, November/December 2004, pp. 108-109, available at [http://content.healthaffairs. org/cgi/reprint/23/6/107.pdf].)

[35] For example, Sherman Folland et al., *The Economics of Health and Health Care*, Prentice-Hall, Upper Saddle River, New Jersey, second edition, 1997, p. 602. For sometime, it has been questioned whether the increased care resulting from reduced out-of-pocket payments from insurance always results in a welfare loss (for example, see Mark Pauly, "More on Moral Hazard," *Journal of Health Economics* 2, 1983, pp. 83-84), going so far as to say that sometimes moral hazard may represent a welfare *gain* to society (see, for example, John A. Nyman, "Is 'Moral Hazard' Inefficient? The Policy Implications of a New Theory," *Health Affairs*, vol 23, no. 5, September/October 2004, pp. 194-199, available at [http://content.healthaffairs.org/cgi/ reprint/23/5/194.pdf]). It should also be noted that the presence of insurance can lead to increased spending for reasons besides individuals' immediate response to potential out-of-pocket costs. For example, insurance may enable providers to charge higher prices, ultimately because individuals are insulated from the true costs (see Folland, p. 246, and Roger K. Howe, "Moral Hazard Health Spending," *Health Affairs*, vol. 24, no. 2, pp. 567-8, available at [http://content.healthaffairs.org/cgi/reprint/ 24/2/568.pdf].

[36] Elizabeth Docteur et al., "The US Health System," available at [http://www.oecdwash. org/PDFILES/us_health_ecowp350.pdf], p. 5.

[37] Nicole Tapay and Fracesca Colombo, "Private Health Insurance in the Netherlands: A Case Study," OECD Health Working Paper No. 18, p. 11, available at [http://www.oecd.org/ dataoecd/19/57/34081266.pdf].

[38] Elizabeth Docteur et al., "The US Health System," available at [http://www. oecdwash. org/PDFILES/us_health_ecowp350.pdf], p. 6.

[39] Elizabeth Docteur, "Reforming Health Systems in OECD Countries," presentation at OECD Breakfast Series, Washington, DC, June 26, 2003, available at [http://www.oecdwash.org/PDFILES/health2003_wash.pdf].

[40] This does not include premiums or tax payments for health insurance. This refers to the cost of actual health care services paid by individuals.

[41] Information on some European countries' cost-sharing in their public health insurance programs is in Table 7.1 of "Funding Health Care: Options for Europe," World Health Organization, Open University Press: Buckingham (U.K.), 2002, available at [http://www.euro.who.int/document/e74485.pdf]. It is worth noting that high rates of cost-sharing do not always result in low total health spending. For example, Switzerland has the fourth-highest rate of cost-sharing and the third-highest total health spending per capita.

[42] Richer benefit selection and increased health care consumption may or may not be beneficial to individuals. Exploring this is not the intent of this section, but normative questions regarding health care spending are discussed later.

[43] For additional detail, see CRS Report RL33505, *Tax Benefits for Health Insurance and Expenses: Overview of Current Law and Legislation*, by Bob Lyke and Julie M. Whittaker.

[44] U.S. Office of Management and Budget, "Tax Expenditures," in *Budget of the United States Government 2008, Analytical Perspectives*, p. 289, available at [http://www.whitehouse.gov/omb/budget/fy2008/pdf/apers/receipts.pdf]. U.S. population on July 1, 2006 was 299,398,484. Table 1: Annual Estimates of the Population for the United States, Regions, and States and for Puerto Rico: April 1, 2000 to July 1, 2006 (NST-EST2006-01), Population Division, U.S. Census Bureau, December 22, 2006, available at [http://www.census.gov/popest/states/tables/NST-EST2006-01.xls].

[45] Total tax expenditures are from "Estimates of Federal Tax Expenditures for Fiscal Years 2006-2010," Joint Committee on Taxation, U.S. Government Printing Office, April 25, 2006, available at [http://www.house.gov/jct/s-2-06.pdf].

[46] "For example, Hispanic women, particularly Mexican, bring with them a cultural belief that certain parts of their body should only be touched by their husbands. However, if this cultural belief causes a woman to refuse a breast or pelvic examination, then we must work with her to adopt new beliefs so that these examinations help her maintain good health." From Lynette Grouse, "Reducing Disparities in Cancer Health Care," *BenchMarks*, November 30, 2005, vol. 5, no. 6.

[47] Minah Kim, Robert Blendon, and John Benson, "How Interested Are Americans In New Medical Technologies? A Multicountry Comparison," *Health Affairs*, September/October 2001, vol. 20, no. 5, pp. 194-200, available at [http://content.healthaffairs.org/cgi/reprint/ 20/5/194.pdf].

[48] From custom data table on the website of The Dartmouth Atlas of Health Care [http://www.dartmouthatlas.org/data_tools.shtm], using hospital referral regions. Dartmouth researchers have published much research on the geographic variation in Medicare spending. Regarding the south Florida phenomena, see the previously cited article by Jonathan Skinner and John E. Wennberg, "Exceptionalism Or Extravagance?"

[49] John Wennberger et al., The Center for Evaluative Clinical Sciences, Dartmouth Medical School, *The Quality of Medical Care in the United States: A Report on the Medicare Program, The Dartmouth Atlas of Health Care 1999* (Chicago: Health Forum, Inc., 1999), available at [http://www.dartmouthatlas.org/atlases/99Atlas.pdf], p. 11. Gina Kolata, "Patients in Florida Lining Up For All That Medicare Covers," *New York Times*, September 13, 2003, p. A1.

[50] IMS Management Consulting [David Gascoigne], "DTC at the Crossroads: A 'Direct' Hit ... or Miss?" *IMS Issues and Insights*, September 23, 2004, at [http://www.imshealth.com/ims/portal/front/articleC/0,2777,6599_5266_58193110,00.html].

[51] Meredith B. Rosenthal, Ernst R. Berndt, Julie M. Donohue, Arnold M. Epstein, and Richard G. Frank, *Demand Effects of Recent Changes in Prescription Drug Promotion* (Menlo Park, CA: The Kaiser Family Foundation, June 2003), pp. 18-19.

[52] New Zealand is the other industrialized country that allows direct-to-consumer advertising of prescription drugs.

[53] Gerard Anderson, testimony to the House Energy and Commerce Subcommittee on Oversight and Investigations, June 24, 2004.

[54] Anderson et al., "It's the Prices, Stupid," p. 102.

[55] Cara S. Lesser and Paul B. Ginsburg, "Update on the Nation's Health Care System: 1997-1999," *Health Affairs*, November/December 2000, vol. 19, no. 6, pp. 206-216, available at [http://content.healthaffairs.org/cgi/reprint/19/6/206.pdf].

[56] "UnitedHealth Group Completes Merger with PacifiCare Health Systems, Inc.," UnitedHealth Group news release, December 21, 2005, available at [http://www.unitedhealthgroup.com/news/rel2005/1221PHS.htm].

[57] James C. Robinson, "Consolidation and the Transformation of Competition in Health Insurance," *Health Affairs*, November/December 2004, vol. 23, no. 6, pp. 11-24, available at [http://content.healthaffairs.org/cgi/reprint/23/6/11.pdf.]

[58] Sherman Folland et al., The Economics of Health and Health Care, p. 605.

[59] "Preference-Sensitive Care," A Dartmouth Atlas Project Topic Brief, November 15, 2005, available at [http://www.dartmouthatlas.org/topics/preference_sensitive.pdf].

[60] "Supply-Sensitive Care," A Dartmouth Atlas Project Topic Brief, November 14, 2005, available at [http://www.dartmouthatlas.org/topics/ supply_sensitive.pdf].

[61] Ibid.

[62] Barbara Starfield et al., "The Effects Of Specialist Supply On Populations' Health: Assessing The Evidence," *Health Affairs,* Web exclusive, March 15, 2005, pp. W5-97-107, available at [http://content.healthaffairs.org/ cgi/reprint/hlthaff.w5.97v1.pdf].

[63] For angioplasties, the growth in procedures was driven by increased utilization by comparatively healthy patients who did not have acute myocardial infarction. Brahmajee Nallamothu, Mary Rogers, Michael Chernew, et al., "Opening of Specialty Cardiac Hospitals and Use of Coronary Revascularization in Medicare Beneficiaries," *JAMA - The Journal of the American Medical Association,* March 7, 2007, vol. 297, no. 9, pp. 962-968, available at [http://jama.ama-assn.org/cgi/content/abstract/297/9/962].

[64] The R-squared is 0.94, among 25 reporting countries.

[65] E. Van Doorslaer, X. Koolman, and F. Puffer, "Equity in the Use of Physician Visits in OECD Countries: Has Equal Treatment for Equal Need Been Achieved?" in *Measuring Up: Improving Health System Performance in OECD Countries* (Paris: Organization for Economic Coooperation and Development, 2002), pp. 225-248.

[66] Barbara Starfield, Leiyu Shi, Atul Grover, et al., "The Effects Of Specialist Supply On Populations' Health: Assessing The Evidence," *Health Affairs*, Web exclusive, March 15, 2005, pp. W5-97-W5-107, available at [http://content.healthaffairs.org/ cgi/reprint/hlthaff. w5.97v1.pdf].

[67] Katherine Baicker and Amitabh Chandra, "Medicare Spending, the Physician Workforce, and Beneficiaries' Quality of Care," *Health Affairs*, Web exclusive, April 7, 2004, pp. W4-184-W4-197, available at [http://content.healthaffairs.org/cgi/reprint/hlthaff.w4.184v1.pdf].

[68] W. Pete Welch, Diana Verrilli, Steven Katz, et al., "A Detailed Comparison of Physician Services for the Elderly in the United States and Canada," *JAMA - The Journal of the American Medical Association,* May 8, 1996, vol. 275, no. 18, pp. 1410-1416.

[69] Michael Gusmano, Victor Rodwin, and Daniel Weisz, "A New Way To Compare Health Systems: Avoidable Hospital Conditions In Manhattan And Paris," *Health Affairs*, March/April 2006, vol. 25, no. 2, pp. 510-520, available at [http://content.healthaffairs.org/ cgi/reprint/25/2/510].

[70] David Studdert, Michelle Mello, William Sage, et al., "Defensive Medicine Among High-Risk Specialist Physicians in a Volatile Malpractice Environment," *JAMA - The Journal of the American Medical Association*, June

1, 2005, vol. 293, pp. 2609-2617, available at [http://jama.ama-assn.org/cgi/content/short/293/21/2609].

[71] Daniel Kessler and Mark McClellan, "Do doctors practice defensive medicine?" *The Quarterly Journal of Economics*, May 1996, vol. 111, no. 2, pp. 353-390, available at [http://www.jstor.org/view/00335533/di976354/97p00433/0].

[72] Perry Beider and Stuart Hagen, "Limiting Tort Liability for Medical Malpractice," Congressional Budget Office, January 8, 2004, available at [http://www.cbo.gov/ ftpdocs/49xx/doc4968/01-08-MedicalMalpractice.pdf].

[73] Chapin White and Stuart Hagen, "Medical Malpractice Tort Limits and Health Care Spending," Background Paper, Congressional Budget Office, April 2006, available at [http://www.cbo.gov/ftpdocs/71xx/doc7174/04-28-Medical Malpractice.pdf], p. 3.

[74] Alison Evans Cuellar and Paul J. Gertler, "How the Expansion of Hospital Systems Has Affected Consumers," *Health Affairs*, January/February 2005, vol. 24, no. 1, pp. 213-219, available at [http://content.healthaffairs.org/cgi/reprint/24/1/213.pdf]; Cory Capps and David Dranove, "Hospital Consolidation and Negotiated PPO Prices," *Health Affairs*, March/April 2004, vol. 23, no. 2, pp. 175-181, available at [http://content.healthaffairs.org/ cgi/reprint/23/2/175.pdf].

[75] George Trefgarne, "NHS reachs 1.4m employees," U.K. *Telegraph*, March 23, 2005, [http://www.telegraph.co.uk/money/main.jhtml?xml=/money/2005/03/23/cnnhs 23.xml].

[76] Elizabeth Docteur, "Reforming Health Systems in OECD Countries," presentation at OECD Breakfast Series, Washington, DC, June 26, 2003, available at [http://www.oecdwash.org/PDFILES/health2003_wash.pdf].

[77] Simon Stevens, "Reform Strategies for the English NHS," *Health Affairs*, May/June 2004, vol. 23, no. 6, pp. 37-44, available at [http://content.healthaffairs.org/cgi/reprint/ 23/3/37.pdf].

[78] Steffie Woolhandler et al., "Costs of Health Care Administration in the United States and Canada," *New England Journal of Medicine*, August 21, 2003, vol. 349, no. 8, p. 768.

[79] Henry J. Aaron, "The costs of health care administration in the United States and Canada -questionable answers to a questionable question," *The New England Journal of Medicine,* August 21, 2003, vol. 349, no. 8, p. 801, available at [http://content.nejm.org/cgi/ content/extract/349/8/801].

[80] Peter S. Hussey, Gerard F. Anderson, Robin Osborn, et al., "How Does The Quality of Care Compare in Five Countries?" *Health Affairs,* May/June 2004, vol. 23, no. 3, pp. 89-99, available at [http://content.healthaffairs.org/cgi/reprint/23/3/89].

[81] Karen Davis, Cathy Schoen, Stephen Schoenbaum, et al., "Mirror, Mirror on the Wall: An Update on the Quality of American Health Care through the

Patient's Lens," The Commonwealth Fund, April 2006, available at [http://www.cmwf.org/usr_doc/Davis_ mirrormirror_915.pdf].

[82] Karen Davis et al., "Mirror, Mirror on the Wall: An International Update on the Comparative Performance of American Health Care," The Commonwealth Fund, May 2007, [http://www.commonwealthfund.org/usr_doc/ Davis_ mirrormirrorinternationalpdate_ 1027.pdf?section=4039].

[83] Wait times are also reported to be low in Austria, Belgium, France, Germany, Japan, Luxembourg, and Switzerland. Conversely, wait times are a serious health policy issue in Australia, Canada, Denmark, Finland, Ireland, Italy, the Netherlands, New Zealand, Norway, Spain, Sweden, and the United Kingdom. Luigi Siciliani and Jeremy Hurst, "OECD Health Working Papers No. 7: Explaining Waiting Times Variations for Elective Surgery across OECD Countries," Organization for Economics Cooperation and Development, 2003, available at [http://www.oecd.org/dataoecd/ 31/10/17256025.pdf].

[84] R.J. Blendon et al., "Inequities in Health Care: A Five-Country Survey," *Health Affairs,* May/June 2002, vol. 21, no. 3, pp. 182-191, available at [http://content.healthaffairs.org/ cgi/reprint/21/3/182].

[85] Luigi Siciliani and Jeremy Hurst, "OECD Health Working Papers No. 7: Explaining Waiting Times Variations for Elective Surgery across OECD Countries," Organization for Economics Cooperation and Development, 2003, available at [http://www.oecd.org/ dataoecd/31/10/17256025.pdf].

[86] Cathy Schoen, Robin Osborn, Phuong Trang Huynh, et al., "Primary Care And Health System Performance: Adults' Experiences in Five Countries," *Health Affairs,* Web exclusive, October 28, 2004, pp. W4-487-W4-503, available at [http://content. healthaffairs.org/cgi/reprint/hlthaff.w4.487v1.pdf]; Karen Davis, Cathy Schoen, Stephen Schoenbaum, et al., "Mirror, Mirror on the Wall: An Update on the Quality of American Health Care through the Patient's Lens," The Commonwealth Fund, April 2006, available at [http://www.cmwf.org/ usr_doc/Davis_ mirrormirror_915.pdf].

[87] There appears to be no relationship between the proportion of a country's population that is elderly and the percentage of the population that reports being in "good" or better health.

[88] For more information, see CRS Report RL32792, *Life Expectancy in the United States,* by Laura Shrestha.

[89] Heart diseases include ischemic heart diseases, acute myocardial infarction, and cerebrovascular diseases. Respiratory diseases include influenza, pneumonia, bronchitis, asthma, and emphysema.

[90] Karen Davis, Cathy Schoen, Stephen Schoenbaum, et al., "Mirror, Mirror on the Wall: An Update on the Quality of American Health Care through the Patient's Lens," The Commonwealth Fund, April 2006, available at [http://www.cmwf.org/usr_doc/Davis_ mirrormirror_915.pdf].

[91] A 1990 analysis that added late fetal deaths in its calculation of infant mortality rates found that the United States was ranked 10th out of 13 countries on this measure. This is only slightly better than the United States' rank using the more traditional methodology, which resulted in a rating of 13th out of 13 countries. U.S. Congress, Office of Technology Assessment, *International Health Statistics: What the Numbers Mean for the United States — Background Paper*, OTA-BP-H-116 (Washington, DC: U.S. Government Printing Office, November 1993), available at [http://www.wws.princeton.edu/ota/disk1/ 1994/9418/9418.PDF], pp. 31, 35, 46.

[92] David M. Cutler and Mark McClellan, "Is Technological Change In Medicine Worth It?" *Health Affairs*, September/October 2001, vol. 20, no. 5, pp. 11-29, available at [http://content.healthaffairs.org/cgi/reprint/20/5/11].

[93] David M. Cutler, Allison B. Rosen, and Sandeep Vijan, "The Value of Medical Spending in the United States, 1960-2000," *The New England Journal of Medicine*, August 31, 2006, vol. 355, no. 9, p. 920, available at [http://content.nejm.org/ cgi/content/abstract/355/9/920], subscription required. Cutler and colleagues find that each year of life expectancy gains costs more than the last — the gain of an additional year of life expectancy cost $7,400 in the 1970s, but the most recent additional year cost $36,300 in the 1990s.

[94] Ibid, p. 924.

[95] See, for example: Elliott S. Fisher et al., "The Implications of Regional Variations in Medicare Spending. Part 1: The Content, Quality, and Accessibility of Care," *Annals of Internal Medicine*, February 18, 2003, vol. 138, pp. 273-287, available at [http://www.annals.org/cgi/reprint/ 138/4/ 273.pdf]. Patients received 60% more care in some regions, yet had a similar baseline health status as patients in lower-spending regions.

[96] Victor R. Fuchs, "More Variation In Use of Care, More Flat-Of-The-Curve Medicine," *Health Affairs*, Web exclusive, October 2, 2004, pp. VAR-104-VAR-107, available at [http://content.healthaffairs.org/cgi/reprint/ hlthaff. var.104v1]; Katherine Baicker and Amitabh Chandra, "Medicare Spending, The Physician Workforce, And Beneficiaries' Quality of Care," *Health Affairs*, Web exclusive, April 7, 2004, pp. W4-184-W4-197, available at [http://content. healthaffairs.org/cgi/reprint/hlthaff.w4.184v1].

[97] Victor R. Fuchs, "More Variation In Use of Care, More Flat-Of-The-Curve Medicine," *Health Affairs*, Web exclusive, October 2, 2004, pp. VAR-104-VAR-107, available at [http://content.healthaffairs.org/cgi/reprint/hlthaff.var.104v1]. See also Uwe Reinhardt, "Variations in California Hospital Regions: Another Wake-Up Call For Sleeping Policymakers," *Health Affairs*, Web exclusive, November 16, 2005, pp. W5-549-W5-551, available at [http://content.healthaffairs.org/ cgi/reprint/hlthaff.w5.549v1?ck=nck].

[98] Richard Kronick and Todd Gilmer, "Explaining The Decline in Health Insurance Coverage, 1979-2005," *Health Affairs*, vol. 18, no. 2, March/April 1999, available at [http://content.healthaffairs.org/cgi/reprint/18/2/30].

[99] Excess growth is defined by this researcher as "the rate of increase in real health spending per capita above and beyond the increase attributable to economic growth and population aging."

[100] Chapin White, "Health Care Spending Growth: How Different Is The United States From The Rest Of The OECD?" *Health Affairs*, January/February 2007, vol. 26, no. 1, pp. 154-161, available at [http://content.healthaffairs.org/cgi/reprint/26/1/154], subscription required. White is a CBO analyst, but his views do not necessarily reflect those of CBO.

[101] National Health Expenditures by type of service and source of funds, CY 1960-2005, National Health Expenditure Data, Centers for Medicare and Medicaid Services, available at [http://www.cms.hhs.gov/NationalHealthExpendData/02_NationalHealthAccounts Historical.asp].

[102] Association of American Medical Colleges, "2006 Medical School Graduation Questionnaire: All Schools Report, FINAL," p. 49, available at [http://www.aamc.org/ data/gq/allschoolsreports/2006.pdf].

INDEX

A

access, x, 2, 104
accidents, 91
accounting, 9, 35, 115
acquired immunodeficiency syndrome (AIDS), x, 2, 55, 91
acquisitions, 70
adjusted gross income (AGI), 65
administration, 50, 52, 70, 80, 113, 133
advertising, 67, 131
age, 29, 55, 57, 67, 89, 91, 94, 101, 103
aging, 56, 57, 104, 136
aging population, 57
alcohol, 55, 56
alcohol consumption, 56
aneurysm, 42, 127
angina, 10
angioplasties, ix, 1, 19, 22, 23, 126, 132
artery, 19, 22, 23, 42, 127
arthroplasty, 41
assumptions, 31
asthma, 134
attitudes, 67
Australia, 3, 34, 36, 37, 81, 85, 94, 100, 119, 121, 127, 134
Austria, 3, 94, 134
authority, 104

B

bargaining, 69, 79
Belgium, 3, 4, 5, 6, 10, 16, 26, 27, 34, 36, 46, 47, 50, 51, 92, 93, 94, 134
beliefs, 130
benefits, 52, 65, 103
birth(s), 89, 94, 99, 101
blood flow, 10
bone, 126
bone marrow, 126
brain, 10
brand name drugs, 44, 111
breakdown, 50
breast, 81, 119, 130
breast cancer, 81, 119
Britain, 79
bronchitis, 134
bypass graft, 19, 22, 23, 42, 126, 127

C

caesarean section, 18
California, 135
calorie, 55
Canada, 3, 4, 5, 6, 10, 11, 34, 36, 41, 42, 43, 45, 46, 56, 69, 75, 80, 81, 82, 85, 87, 89, 92, 93, 94, 100, 101, 115, 119, 121, 126, 127, 132, 133, 134

Canberra, 128
cancer, x, 2, 55, 73, 81, 91, 119
cancer screening, 81
capacity, 73, 74, 85
cardiac catheterization, 126
Census Bureau, 130
cerebrovascular diseases, 10, 134
cervical cancer, 81
Chicago, 131
childbirth, 13, 15
children, 101
chronic illness, 73
clinics, 11, 125
cohort, 103
commercial, 70
commodities, ix, 1, 31
compensation, 34, 36
competition, 19
complexity, 52
complications, 83
components, 31, 49, 53
congestive heart failure, 73
Congress, 135
Congressional Budget Office (CBO), 77, 104, 133, 136
Congressional Research Service (CRS), 4, 6, 24, 25, 34, 36, 50, 125, 130, 134
consolidation, 69, 79
consulting, 67
consumers, 53
consumption, 45, 55, 56, 117, 127, 128, 130
consumption patterns, 127, 128
control, 15, 79
conversion, 31, 127
coronary artery bypass graft, 19, 22, 23, 42, 127
coronary bypasses, ix, 1
correlation, 74
costs, 33, 41, 42, 49, 50, 52, 56, 61, 62, 65, 69, 70, 75, 80, 103, 104, 129, 133, 135
coverage, 61, 62, 65, 104
covering, 32, 61
cross-country, 74, 127
CT scan, 19, 26, 39, 109
culture, 67

currency, 4, 31, 44, 127
Czech Republic, 3, 4, 5, 6, 34, 35, 36, 46, 47, 50, 92, 93, 94

D

Dartmouth College, 29
death rate, 91
death(s), 75, 91, 94, 97, 101, 123, 129, 135
debt(s), 33, 115
decisions, 44, 127
definition, 126
delivery, ix, 1, 15, 79
demand, 53, 59, 61, 67, 71, 73, 74
demographic characteristics, 91
demographic factors, 75
demographics, 3
Denmark, 3, 4, 5, 6, 10, 34, 36, 37, 46, 82, 92, 93, 94, 95, 100, 101, 105, 134
desire, 53
diabetes, 55
diabetic, 81, 119
diet, 55
direct-to-consumer (DTC), 67, 131
discharges, 9, 125
distribution, 62
divergence, 41
dividends, 52
doctor(s), ix, x, 1, 2, 7, 9, 11, 21, 31, 33, 53, 73, 75, 79, 81, 83, 85, 97, 100, 109, 119, 121, 125, 133
doctor visits, ix, 1, 9, 11, 21, 31, 85, 109, 121, 125
drinking, 117
drugs, 10, 43, 44, 45, 67, 111, 128, 131

E

economic growth, 104, 136
economic theory, 33
economics, 61
education, 33
elderly, 16, 75, 117, 134
election, 127

Index   139

elective surgery, 85
emphysema, 134
employees, 49, 133
employment, 129
end-of-life care, 29
England, 133, 135
equipment, 19, 31, 39, 79, 109
Europe, 69, 80, 130
European, 9, 128, 130
evidence, 18
examinations, 130
exchange rates, 31, 44, 127
expansions, 19
expenditures, 50, 65, 80, 107, 128, 130

F

failure, 73
fat, 128
fetal death, 135
finance, 4, 5, 6
financing, 79, 104
Finland, 3, 34, 94, 101, 105, 134
flat-of-the-curve medicine, 103
food, 55
France, 3, 4, 5, 6, 11, 34, 45, 46, 80, 91, 92, 93, 94, 100, 134
fruits, 128
funds, 136

G

GDP, 2, 3, 4, 6, 34, 35, 36, 59, 79, 80, 107, 115, 128
GDP per capita, 2, 35, 128
general practitioner, 33, 34, 36, 75, 79, 109, 115
generic drugs, 43, 44, 111
Germany, 3, 10, 11, 34, 57, 61, 80, 94, 115, 119, 134
goods and services, 31, 32, 53
government, 52, 69, 79, 103, 127
Government Accountability Office (GAO), 43, 127

Greece, 3, 4, 5, 6, 10, 11, 16, 26, 27, 34, 35, 36, 50, 56, 82, 92, 93, 94, 100
growth, 34, 36, 73, 104, 105, 132, 136
gynecologists, 77

H

Harvard, 129
head, 126
health, ix, x, 1, 2, 3, 4, 5, 7, 9, 10, 13, 15, 19, 29, 31, 32, 33, 34, 35, 36, 39, 45, 49, 50, 52, 53, 55, 56, 57, 59, 61, 62, 65, 67, 69, 70, 71, 73, 74, 75, 77, 79, 80, 81, 85, 87, 89, 91, 92, 103, 104, 107, 113, 115, 119, 123, 126, 128, 129, 130, 133, 134, 135, 136
health care, ix, x, 1, 2, 3, 4, 7, 9, 10, 13, 15, 19, 29, 31, 32, 33, 39, 45, 49, 50, 52, 53, 55, 56, 57, 59, 61, 62, 65, 67, 69, 70, 71, 73, 74, 75, 79, 80, 81, 85, 87, 89, 91, 103, 104, 107, 113, 115, 119, 123, 128, 130, 133
health care costs, 33, 62, 65
health care professionals, 33, 115
health care system, 32, 61, 80, 81, 85, 91, 123
health expenditure, 4, 5, 49, 107
health insurance, 52, 61, 65, 69, 70, 80, 104, 130
Health Savings Accounts, 65
health services, 34, 36, 69, 79
health status, 87, 92, 123, 129, 135
heart, 7, 10, 13, 15, 17, 19, 55, 69, 73, 77, 85, 91, 109, 126, 134
heart attack, 7, 10, 15, 69
heart disease, 55, 77, 91, 134
heart failure, 73
hepatitis B, 81
higher education, 33
hip, 19, 41, 85, 126
hip arthroplasty, 41
hip replacement, 19, 126
Hispanic, 130
HMOs, 43
hospital(s), ix, 1, 7, 9, 10, 11, 13, 15, 16, 18, 19, 29, 41, 49, 50, 53, 61, 73, 74, 75, 79, 85, 109, 125, 127, 131
hospital beds, 109

hospital care, 9, 49
hospital stays, 15, 41, 109
hospitalization(s), ix, 1, 9, 15, 19, 31, 73
hospitalized, 69, 83, 125
House, 131
Hungary, 3, 34, 46, 47, 50, 51, 92, 94, 100
hypertension, 129
hypertensive, 10, 81, 119

I

imaging, 19, 50, 73
immunodeficiency, 55
incentives, 74
incidence, x, 2, 55, 57, 91
income, 53, 59, 65, 104, 129
income tax, 65
indicators, 81
industrialized countries, 67, 75
industry, 34, 36
infant mortality rate, 99, 123, 135
infarction, 10, 15, 77, 132, 134
inflation, 35, 104
influenza, 134
infrastructure, 79
insight, ix, x, 2
insurance, 50, 52, 61, 65, 69, 70, 79, 80, 104, 113, 129, 130
intensity, ix, 1, 3, 7, 13, 15, 19, 29, 31, 53, 103
intensive care unit, 125
international standards, 69
introductory prices, 39
investment, 50, 67
Ireland, 3, 11, 34, 50, 87, 92, 93, 94, 100, 105, 134
Italy, 3, 10, 11, 16, 57, 82, 91, 92, 93, 94, 100, 134

J

Japan, 3, 4, 5, 6, 10, 11, 16, 19, 26, 27, 43, 46, 47, 50, 51, 57, 63, 69, 85, 89, 92, 93, 94, 100, 101, 126, 134

Joint Committee on Taxation, 130

K

Kaiser Family Foundation, 131
kidney, 19, 81, 119, 126
kidney transplant, 119
knee replacement, 19, 85, 126
Korea, 3, 10, 11, 16, 82, 92, 93, 94, 100, 101

L

labor, 33, 35
labor-intensive, 33
lead, 19, 31, 55, 62, 73, 129
life expectancy, x, 2, 89, 94, 103, 123, 135
likelihood, 129
litigation, 77
liver, 126
loans, 33
lower prices, 69
lung, 73, 126
lung disease, 73
Luxembourg, ix, 1, 2, 3, 4, 5, 6, 9, 46, 52, 56, 70, 92, 93, 94, 128, 134

M

magnetic resonance imaging (MRI), 19, 27, 109
malpractice, 77
management, 75
Manhattan, 75, 132
manufacturer, 44
market(s), 35, 69, 70
market share, 70
marrow, 126
Massachusetts, 129
measles, 81
measurement, 123, 127
measures, 13, 19, 123
media, 80
median, 19, 22, 23, 49, 50, 52, 113, 126
Medicaid, 43, 56, 69, 129, 136

medical care, ix, 1, 31, 75, 97, 103, 115
medical school, 115
Medicare, 29, 56, 67, 69, 73, 103, 104, 126, 131, 132, 135, 136
medication, 97
medicine, 67, 77, 103, 133
men, 89
Mexico, 3, 10, 16, 34, 62, 92, 94, 99
Miami, 29, 67
models, 104
molecules, 43, 45
money, ix, x, 1, 65, 133
moral hazard, 61, 62, 129
mortality rate, x, 2, 91, 94, 99, 101, 123, 135
myocardial infarction, 10, 15, 77, 132, 134

N

nation, 45, 55, 128
National Health Service (NHS), 79, 80, 133
neoplasms, 55
Netherlands, 3, 4, 5, 6, 16, 34, 36, 46, 47, 50, 61, 82, 92, 93, 94, 129, 134
New England, 133, 135
New Jersey, 129
New York, 128, 131
New York Times, 131
New Zealand, 3, 11, 16, 27, 34, 37, 50, 55, 81, 87, 92, 94, 95, 100, 101, 119, 131, 134
non-emergency, x, 2, 85, 121
Norway, 3, 9, 11, 34, 92, 94, 100, 101, 134
nurses, 19, 24, 25, 33, 34, 35, 36, 79, 109, 115
nursing, 16, 125
nursing home, 16, 125

O

obesity, x, 2, 55, 56
obstetricians, 77
Office of Management and Budget, 130
organ, 19, 109, 126
organization, 103
Organization for Economic Cooperation and Development (OECD), ix, x, 1, 2, 3, 4, 5, 6, 9, 10, 11, 15, 16, 17, 18, 19, 21, 22, 23, 24, 25, 26, 27, 31, 33, 34, 35, 36, 37, 39, 41, 45, 46, 47, 49, 50, 51, 52, 53, 55, 56, 57, 59, 61, 62, 63, 65, 67, 74, 75, 79, 81, 82, 85, 87, 89, 91, 92, 93, 94, 97, 99, 100, 101, 103, 104, 105, 107, 109, 111, 113, 115, 117, 125, 126, 128, 129, 130, 132, 133, 134, 136
outliers, 2
out-of-pocket, 61, 65, 104, 113, 129
outpatient, 9, 11, 21, 49, 50, 109, 117, 125
over-the-counter, 43, 45
overweight, 55, 117

P

pacemakers, 126
Paris, 75, 132
patients, 7, 9, 11, 13, 16, 41, 53, 71, 73, 74, 81, 83, 100, 103, 104, 119, 125, 132, 135
peers, 67
Pennsylvania, 77
per capita, ix, 1, 2, 3, 4, 5, 9, 10, 11, 19, 21, 31, 35, 39, 49, 50, 56, 57, 59, 74, 85, 89, 92, 93, 109, 111, 117, 125, 128, 130, 136
perinatal, 125
personal, 50, 65
pharmaceutical(s), 45, 49, 53, 67, 128
pharmaceutical companies, 53
physicians, 11, 29, 35, 37, 49, 50, 73, 75, 77, 79, 85, 109, 121, 125, 132
pneumonia, 134
Poland, 3, 34, 94, 100
policy makers, 80
poor, 97, 129
population, x, 2, 9, 11, 13, 19, 23, 52, 53, 55, 57, 61, 67, 75, 79, 87, 91, 104, 109, 117, 123, 125, 126, 130, 134, 136
Portugal, 3, 4, 5, 6, 16, 26, 27, 34, 46, 55, 91, 92, 93, 94, 100
power, 4, 5, 31, 34, 36, 41, 46, 50, 51, 69, 79, 92, 93, 127
PPO, 133
preference, 131
premature babies, 99, 101

premature death, 91, 94
premiums, 52, 65, 104, 130
prevention, 49
price effect, 70
prices, ix, 1, 31, 39, 41, 42, 43, 44, 53, 59, 67, 69, 79, 104, 115, 127, 129
primary care, 11, 73, 75, 85, 121, 125
problem drinking, 56
process indicators, 81
production, 33, 39, 104
profession(s), 33, 34, 36
profits, 52
program, 61, 103
prostatectomy, 126
protein, 128
public financing, 79
public health, 49, 50, 61, 80, 130
Puerto Rico, 130
purchasing power, 4, 5, 31, 34, 36, 41, 46, 50, 51, 92, 93, 127
purchasing power parity(ies) (PPPs), 31, 44, 92, 127

R

race, 29
radiologists, 77
RAND Health Insurance Experiment, 61, 129
reduction, 129
reforms, 77, 104
relationship, 2, 73, 77, 134
repair, 42, 127
reserves, 52
resources, x, 2, 13
respiratory, 91
responsiveness, 104
returns, 65, 67
revascularization, 23, 132
revenue, 44, 127
rice, 31
R-squared, 6, 36, 92, 93, 132

S

sales, 44, 45, 127
sample, 127
savings, 77
scarcity, 35
school, 33, 115
self-employed, 35, 36, 65
sex, 29
sharing, 61, 62, 129, 130
sites, 79
skills, 35
smokers, 56
smoking, 56, 117
society, 129
Spain, 3, 4, 5, 6, 10, 11, 16, 46, 82, 92, 93, 94, 100, 134
specialists, 11, 33, 34, 35, 36, 73, 75, 79, 109, 115, 125
standards, 69
stereotype, 80
strategies, 69
sugar, 56, 117
suppliers, 53
supply, 35, 53, 59, 70, 71, 73, 75, 79, 109, 132
surgeons, 77
surgery(ies), x, 2, 7, 13, 41, 42, 73, 74, 80, 85, 100, 121, 126, 127, 134
survival, 81, 99, 101, 119
survival rate, 81, 119
Sweden, 3, 4, 5, 6, 11, 34, 36, 37, 46, 49, 56, 92, 93, 94, 100, 101, 134
Switzerland, ix, 1, 3, 4, 5, 6, 9, 11, 34, 36, 46, 91, 92, 93, 94, 130, 134
syndrome, 55
systems, 69, 79, 80, 81, 123

T

tax policy, 65
tax preferences, 65
teaching, 41
technology, 19
theory, 33

time, 29, 73, 81, 83, 85, 99, 104, 119, 126
tobacco, 55
tort reforms, 77
training, 35
transplant, 13, 81, 119
transport, 50
trend, 35
Turkey, 3, 16, 26, 37, 46, 47, 50, 51, 57, 62, 92, 94, 99

U

U.S. economy, ix, 1, 2
uninsured, x, 2, 61, 62, 69
United Kingdom, 3, 19, 34, 43, 45, 50, 51, 55, 79, 81, 85, 92, 93, 94, 100, 119, 121, 127, 134
United States, ix, x, 1, 2, 3, 7, 9, 10, 11, 15, 18, 19, 21, 29, 33, 34, 35, 36, 39, 41, 42, 43, 44, 45, 49, 50, 52, 53, 55, 56, 57, 59, 61, 62, 65, 67, 69, 70, 75, 79, 80, 81, 82, 85, 87, 89, 91, 93, 94, 97, 99, 100, 101, 103, 104, 105, 107, 109, 111, 113, 115, 117, 119, 121, 123, 125, 126, 127, 128, 129, 130, 131, 132, 133, 134, 135, 136
universality, 62

V

variation, 2, 29, 59, 62, 73, 129, 131
vegetables, 128

W

wages, 34, 36, 65
wait times, x, 2, 85, 121, 134
waiting times, 85
Washington, 130, 133, 135
wealth, 35
welfare loss, 129
wholesale, 44, 127
women, 13, 89, 130
workers, 34, 35, 36, 65
World Health Organization, 130